THE
HASHIMOTO'S THYROIDITIS
Healing Diet

A Complete Program for Eating Smart,
Reversing Symptoms and Feeling Great

Kate Barrington

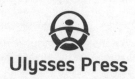

Ulysses Press

Published in the United States by:
Ulysses Press
P.O. Box 3440
Berkeley, CA 94703
www.ulyssespress.com

ISBN13: 978-1-61243-596-1
Library of Congress Control Number: 2016934494

Printed in the United States by United Graphics
10 9 8 7 6 5 4 3 2 1

Acquisitions Editor: Casie Vogel
Managing Editor: Claire Chun
Project Editor: Alice Riegert
Editor: Susan Lang
Proofreader: Lauren Harrison
Index: Jay Kreider
Front cover design: Rebecca Lown
Interior design and layout: what!design @ whatweb.com
Artwork: cover © Serg64/shutterstock.com, page 14 © Tefi/shutterstock.com

Distributed by Publishers Group West

CONTENTS

CHAPTER 8: DINNER • 109

CHAPTER 9: VEGAN AND VEGETARIAN DISHES • • • • • • • • • • • 131

INTRODUCTION

Many people who suffer from fatigue, hoarse voice, and achy bones and joints assume that it is nothing more than the flu. For people with Hashimoto's disease, however, these symptoms are all too familiar and cannot be eradicated with flu medicine or a bowl of chicken soup. People with Hashimoto's disease experience these symptoms and many more on a daily basis, sometimes to the point where it interferes with their daily lives and their ability to work. For people with Hashimoto's, a serious autoimmune disorder, life can be exhausting and painful—especially since there is no cure for the disease.

Hashimoto's disease, also called Hashimoto's thyroiditis, affects roughly 14 million people in the United States alone—nearly 8 percent of the population. Unfortunately, autoimmune diseases in general are still very poorly understood, despite the fact that nearly 24 million Americans are affected and approximately 90 percent of all hypothyroid disorders can be linked to autoimmune disease.[1] Sadly, there is no cure; an autoimmune disease might go into remission, but it will never truly go away.

If you are suffering from Hashimoto's, you may feel as if there is no hope. Don't worry: Although it is true that the disease cannot be cured, it is also true that there are plenty of ways to manage your condition and to find relief from symptoms. This book will show you how. For example, you'll learn that modern technological advances led to the development of a synthetic thyroid hormone that has proved to be a very effective treatment for Hashimoto's.[2]

Along with taking a synthetic hormone, making changes to your diet is essential in managing Hashimoto's. Increasing your intake of iodine, selenium, and other nutrients can help to reduce chronic inflammation, balance hormone levels, and repair damage to the digestive tract caused by Hashimoto's.[3] Dietary management is simple. For many people, it is as easy as taking a few supplements and eating clean, healthy foods. Certain foods should be avoided as they tend to cause Hashimoto's flare-ups. This book will teach you everything you need to manage your Hashimoto's disease effectively, including synthetic hormone therapy as well as diet and lifestyle changes. It will become your road map to remission, guiding you through the necessary steps to relieve your symptoms.

In this book, you will find in-depth information about Hashimoto's and other autoimmune or thyroid conditions to help you gain a deeper understanding of your disease. The book also has a collection of flavorful recipes for breakfast, lunch, dinner, snacks, and more. By the time you finish reading, you will have a greater understanding of your condition and be better equipped to manage it through healthy food and lifestyle choices. So what are you waiting for? Turn the page and get started on a healthier, happier path!

PART I
UNDERSTANDING HASHIMOTO'S DISEASE

CHAPTER 1
What Is Hashimoto's Disease?

"Hashimoto's disease is the most common cause of hypothyroidism in the United States ... [It] typically progresses slowly over years and causes chronic thyroid damage, leading to a drop in thyroid hormone levels in your blood."

—Mayo Clinic, "Hashimoto's Disease"[4]

Hashimoto's is sometimes difficult for people to understand because it is both a thyroid condition and an autoimmune disease. Also known as chronic lymphocytic thyroiditis or autoimmune thyroiditis, Hashimoto's disease can be very serious. In addition to causing chronic fatigue, weight gain, and pain in the joints and muscles, Hashimoto's can actually physically damage the thyroid, impairing its function. If the resulting damage is not treated properly, the thyroid will no longer be able to produce the hormones the body needs to function and the body's systems will start to shut down. When Hashimoto's is left untreated, complications can be fatal, although this is rare.

This chapter provides an overview of the disease, including key information about risk factors that correlate with Hashimoto's as well as common signs and symptoms of the disease.

OVERVIEW OF HASHIMOTO'S DISEASE

At its most basic level, Hashimoto's is a disease in which the body attacks the thyroid gland, causing it to malfunction. The immune system initiates the attack when, for reasons still being studied, it recognizes the body's own healthy thyroid tissue as a foreign invader. When this happens, the immune system launches a defensive response by producing lymphocytes (or T-cells), a type of white blood cell, which invade the thyroid gland. Inside the thyroid, the lymphocytes destroy the healthy cells, tissues, and blood vessels. The damage caused to the thyroid is slow—this is why people with Hashimoto's may go for years before any obvious symptoms develop.

In addition to destroying healthy thyroid tissue, this immune response triggers chronic inflammation that further damages the thyroid. Although the damage cannot be seen from the outside, it slowly destroys the thyroid from the inside, impairing its ability to produce and utilize essential hormones. The point at which the thyroid is so damaged that it can no longer function normally is when symptoms of hypothyroidism develop. In cases where inflammation is particularly bad, the thyroid may become so enlarged that it is visible as a mass growing in the neck. This mass, called a goiter, is one of the most common early symptoms of Hashimoto's.

WHAT CAUSES HASHIMOTO'S DISEASE?

Hashimoto's is a two-fold condition that involves both the thyroid gland and the immune system. In Hashimoto's patients, the immune system mistakenly identifies thyroid tissue as a foreign invader and attacks the healthy tissue instead of protecting it. This is the causative factor that leads to impaired function and chronic inflammation of the thyroid. When the thyroid becomes inflamed and does not work properly, it fails to produce adequate amounts of key thyroid hormones. These hormones are incredibly important, affecting everything from metabolism and respiration to brain development and nervous system function.

While it is well documented that an autoimmune response can lead to hypothyroidism in Hashimoto's patients, doctors and researchers still do not completely understand exactly how autoimmune diseases like Hashimoto's come about in the first place. Roughly 80 different autoimmune diseases have been identified, many of which present with very similar symptoms. In addition to being difficult to diagnose, autoimmune diseases are tricky to treat because a person can have more than one at a time, and the diseases often fluctuate between periods of remission and flare-ups.[5]

Some potential causes of the autoimmune response leading to Hashimoto's include exposure to chemical or environmental irritants, and certain bacteria or viruses, and the use of certain prescription drugs. Different drugs can increase the risk for developing autoimmune diseases—this is referred to as drug-induced autoimmunity. Drug-induced lupus erythematosus is the most studied example and has been associated with a number of medications including the antihistamine hydralazine and the heart medication procainamide. According to Dr. Nikolas R. Hedberg, a board-certified nutritionist and naturopathic practitioner, infections are among the most commonly overlooked causes of autoimmune disease: "In my clinical experience working with many Hashimoto's patients I have found that the most common underlying cause of Hashimoto's disease is a stealth infection that has been overlooked by both conventional and alternative practitioners."

When microorganisms invade the human body, the result is called an infection and there are different levels of infection that can occur in the body. An active infection produces an acute physiologic response that can be observed and tested with laboratory equipment. When symptoms present at a much more subtle level and persist over a longer period, the infection is called subclinical. One step below subclinical infection is the symptomless carrier state, in which organisms are present in the host's body but are well controlled by the immune system.

Finally, in stealth infection, microorganisms are present in the body, but the immune system doesn't recognize them as a threat and routine laboratory tests cannot detect them. Yet, the undetected microorganisms can secrete minute amounts of toxins and other substances that may damage the body. Because the effects are so subtle, the immune system does not mount a defense and the infection can weaken the body and allow other organisms to invade. If any symptoms do occur, they typically have no obvious connection to symptoms that are normally associated with infection, such as fever, cough, and fatigue. The symptoms that present may include chronic diarrhea, anemia, food intolerance, intensified allergy symptoms, hormone imbalance, and even autoimmune disease.[6]

The connection between certain infections and Hashimoto's disease is still being studied to determine whether stealth infections may be a factor causing the disease. Regardless of whether infections are the primary cause for Hashimoto's, it is undisputed that there are certain biological and lifestyle factors that can increase a person's risk for developing the disease.

RISK FACTORS THAT CORRELATE WITH HASHIMOTO'S

Although the exact causes of Hashimoto's disease, and autoimmune diseases in general, are largely unknown, doctors and researchers have discovered that certain factors increase an individual's risk for developing Hashimoto's. For one thing, the disease tends to manifest in individuals between the ages of 30 and 50. Additionally, the disease is seven times more common in women than in men. Hashimoto's also has a genetic component, as it seems to run in families. Researchers are currently working to identify the specific gene or genes responsible for inheritance of the disease. It is not just familial instances of Hashimoto's that can affect inheritance; family history of any thyroid or autoimmune condition can increase an individual's risk for developing Hashimoto's.[7]

In addition to a family history of autoimmune disease, a preexisting autoimmune condition can greatly increase the risk for developing Hashimoto's. An autoimmune condition is an indication that the immune system is already malfunctioning in some way, and this is what increases the risk for an autoimmune response to attack the thyroid gland. Some of the most common autoimmune disorders that may increase the risk for Hashimoto's include Addison's disease, type 1 diabetes, and rheumatoid arthritis.[8] Anyone who has an autoimmune disease and has not been tested for Hashimoto's should be tested.

Other factors that may increase the risk for developing Hashimoto's or another autoimmune disease include the following:[9]

- Nutritional deficiencies (especially iodine and selenium)

- Stealth, viral, bacterial, or yeast infections

- Foodborne bacterial illness

- Chronic stress, enough to cause adrenal insufficiency

- Trauma, such as surgery or an accident

- Hormonal or immune system changes, such as those caused by pregnancy

Although more research is required, some evidence suggests that certain environmental factors may influence the risk for developing an autoimmune disease. For example, chemicals released into the environment, such as certain pesticides, can contribute to autoimmune conditions. So can certain prescription medications, such as those mentioned on page 7. There is also some evidence to suggest that consuming too much iodine could inhibit the production of thyroid hormone in individuals affected by autoimmune hypothyroidism. In cases where hypothyroidism is not autoimmune-related, an iodine deficiency is more likely to be the cause of thyroid issues.[10]

SIGNS AND SYMPTOMS OF THE DISEASE

One of the most harrowing aspects of Hashimoto's disease is that it can manifest with few to no symptoms at first—this is very common with autoimmune diseases in general. In the early stages, there may be some subtle swelling of the neck and throat, but it is easy to confuse this symptom with the symptoms of more common infections. As Hashimoto's disease progresses, damage to the thyroid continues, and eventually the person develops signs of impaired thyroid function, or hypothyroidism.[11] This may include chronic fatigue, dry skin, and pain or swelling in the joints and muscles.

The type of swelling that commonly signals the onset of Hashimoto's disease is called a goiter, and it is the result of an enlarged thyroid. A goiter typically forms on the front or side of the neck, potentially impacting the ability to swallow. In most cases, goiters start off as painless growths, but they can become large enough to cause discomfort by putting pressure on the lower neck. Additional signs and symptoms of Hashimoto's may include the following:

- Chronic fatigue

- Constipation

- Decreased cold tolerance

- Depression or low mood

- Heavy or abnormal menstrual bleeding in women

- Hoarse voice

- Joint pains and stiffness

- Memory loss

- Muscle aches, pains, and weakness

- Muscle weakness (particularly in the lower extremities)

- Pale, dry, or itchy skin

- Puffy face

- Stiffness in the bones and joints

- Swelling in the knees, hands, and feet

- Unexplained weight gain (average 10 to 20 pounds)

Most of the symptoms connected to Hashimoto's disease are the result of low thyroid hormone levels in the bloodstream. If left untreated, an underactive thyroid hormone can contribute to a number of serious health problems, discussed in detail in the next chapter.

CHAPTER 2
The Effects of Hashimoto's Disease on the Body

"Hypothyroidism is a condition in which the body lacks sufficient thyroid hormone. Since the main purpose of thyroid hormone is to 'run the body's metabolism,' it is understandable that people with this condition will have symptoms associated with a slow metabolism,... Hypothyroidism is more common than you would believe, and millions of people are currently hypothyroid and don't know it."

—James Norman, "Hypothyroidism: Too Little Thyroid Hormone"[12]

Many of the symptoms of Hashimoto's are related to autoimmune activity. For healthy individuals, the immune system is a powerful workforce that helps to protect the body against potentially dangerous invaders like viruses, bacteria, and toxins. The human immune system comprises a vast network of cells, tissues, and organs that all work together to identify and neutralize threats. When it recognizes a foreign invader (called an antigen), it sends out leukocytes (white blood cells) to deal with the problem. For each antigen that invades the body, one of two types of leukocytes called lymphocytes produce specific proteins (called antibodies) that adhere to the antigen and, with the help of other immune cells, destroy it. For more information about autoimmune disease and its effect on the body, see Appendix A.

Although the immune system is essential for protection against disease, for people with Hashimoto's it can be a lethal enemy. In addition to attacking harmful invaders, the immune system turns against healthy tissue in the thyroid gland. A small gland in the lower portion of the neck, the thyroid is an integral part of the human endocrine system. In order to truly understand what Hashimoto's disease is and how it affects the body, you must have a basic understanding of what the thyroid gland does and how hypothyroidism can affect the body. This chapter provides an overview of the thyroid gland and its important role in regulating metabolism, as well as key information about the causes and effects of hypothyroidism. It also presents information about the thyroid-related complications of Hashimoto's disease.

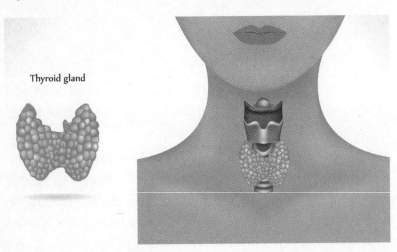

Thyroid gland

WHAT DOES THE THYROID DO IN THE BODY?

The thyroid is part of the endocrine system, which is made up of a network of glands and organs that produce hormones to regulate metabolism, tissue function, growth and development, reproduction, mood, and sleep. The human endocrine system consists of adrenal glands, pituitary gland, thyroid gland, parathyroid glands, pancreas, and ovaries in women or testicles in men.[13]

A gland is a specialized organ that filters certain materials or substances from the blood and processes them, secreting the finished product back into the bloodstream for use throughout the body. Each of the glands that make up the endocrine system plays an important role in regulating certain bodily functions based on the hormones they produce. For example, the pituitary gland, located at the base of the brain in the hypothalamus, is responsible for regulating growth and development—it also plays a role in supporting the function of other endocrine glands. The adrenal glands are located above the kidneys and they produce a number of hormones including adrenaline as well as the steroid hormones cortisol and aldosterone. The hormones produced by the adrenal glands help to regulate metabolism and to suppress autoimmune reactions. Located at the base of the neck, the thyroid gland produces hormones that affect the body's sensitivity to other hormones. It is primarily responsible for helping the body to utilize energy efficiently by regulating body temperature and maintaining the healthy function of the heart, brain, muscles, and other organs.

The thyroid gland produces two different thyroid hormones: triiodothyronine (T3) and thyroxine (T4). Triiodothyronine is the active form of the thyroid hormone; about 20 percent of the body's supply of this hormone is secreted directly into the bloodstream from the thyroid gland itself. The rest of the body's supply of this hormone comes from the conversion of thyroxine into triiodothyronine, which occurs in the kidneys and liver. Thyroxine, also known as a prohormone, has minimal hormonal effect itself, but it can amplify the effects of the active hormone, triiodothyronine.

Although the thyroid produces both T3 and T4, both of these hormones are activated by a hormone produced in the pituitary gland: thyroid-stimulating hormone, or TSH. The relationship between the thyroid and the pituitary gland is described as a "closed-loop" process. When T3 and T4 levels in the blood rise, the pituitary gland lowers production of TSH. When thyroid hormone levels in the bloodstream decrease, TSH production ramps back up. Together, the hormonal response of these two glands helps to regulate the body's metabolism, including heart and digestive functions as well as growth and development.[14]

WHAT IS HYPOTHYROIDISM?

Hypothyroidism is simply the medical term for an underactive thyroid gland. When the thyroid isn't able to produce enough hormone to maintain healthy bodily function, very serious problems can develop. Hypothyroidism affects roughly 4.6 percent of the American population, although many of the people who have this condition are unaware of it. Some of the most common symptoms of hypothyroidism include the following:

- Chronic fatigue

- Constipation

- Decreased cold tolerance

- Depression and/or irritability

- Dry hair and skin

- Heavy or abnormal menstrual cycles in women

- Joint pains and stiffness

- Memory loss

- Puffy face

- Muscle cramps, aches, and weakness

- Slowed heart rate

- Weight gain, difficulty losing weight

These symptoms are the result of inadequate levels of thyroid hormone in the blood. The severity of hypothyroid symptoms is directly influenced by TSH levels. Slightly decreased TSH levels may result in a mild form of hypothyroidism with minimal symptoms. As TSH levels continue to decrease, however, symptoms may become more severe and a change in metabolism may become noticeable.

A number of factors can contribute to the development of hypothyroidism, but the most common cause is Hashimoto's disease. This condition causes the immune system to attack the healthy tissue in the thyroid gland, producing chronic inflammation and inhibiting thyroid function. Thyroiditis is the medical term for inflammation of the thyroid gland; it is also sometimes referred to as the first stage of hypothyroidism. At first, thyroiditis can cause thyroid hormone to leak into the bloodstream, which can lead to hyperthyroidism (increased thyroid hormone levels in the blood). After a month or two, however, thyroiditis typically develops into hypothyroidism.

Although Hashimoto's disease is the most common cause of hypothyroidism, other conditions or factors can contribute to the disease.[15] They include other autoimmune diseases, thyroid surgery, and damage to or abnormalities in the pituitary gland. Hypothyroidism can also be an congenital condition in cases where babies are born without a thyroid gland or with an underdeveloped thyroid gland. The use of certain prescription medications may also impact the function of the thyroid gland, contributing to hypothyroidism.

In most cases, hypothyroidism is a condition that develops slowly, which means that symptoms may go unnoticed for months, or even years. Unfortunately, by the time a diagnosis is made, often the damage to the thyroid gland is very advanced. Treatment at this point is likely a lifetime of hormone replacement therapy.[16]

COMPLICATIONS OF HYPOTHYROIDISM AND HASHIMOTO'S DISEASE

Hashimoto's disease does not always lead to hypothyroidism. In cases of Hashimoto's in which hypothyroidism is not concurrent, symptoms and complications are most commonly due to inflammation in the thyroid resulting from autoimmune activity. Regardless of whether Hashimoto's is concurrent with hypothyroidism, these diseases can lead to serious complications if left untreated or improperly managed.[17] These complications may include:

AUTOIMMUNE DISEASE — For anyone who already has an autoimmune disease (like Hashimoto's), the risk for developing another autoimmune disease is much higher. Some of the diseases most likely to develop concurrent with Hashimoto's are Addison's disease, Graves' disease, type 1 diabetes, pernicious anemia, rheumatoid arthritis, and vitiligo.

THYROID LYMPHOMA — Long-term thyroid damage like that caused by Hashimoto's can increase the risk for a type of thyroid cancer called thyroid lymphoma. This is a rare complication, but it is highly treatable and very curable if caught early.

HEART DISEASE — Thyroid hormone plays a role in regulating a number of important bodily functions including cardiovascular function. The amount of the thyroid hormone thyroxine (T4) in the blood can affect heart rate which, in turn, can affect the healthy function of the heart. High levels of T4 can lead to rapid heart rate while low T4 levels (often caused by hypothyroidism) can slow the heart rate. Low heart rate can lead to a drop in blood pressure and may also correlate to increased LDL or "bad" cholesterol levels.

MENTAL HEALTH PROBLEMS — In addition to regulating physical growth and development, the thyroid gland plays a role in mental health and development. Mild hypothyroidism has been linked to mild forms of depression, which can worsen without treatment. Long-term Hashimoto's disease and/or hypothyroidism can also lead to slowed cognitive performance, memory loss, and symptoms of psychosis such as auditory and visual hallucinations.

SEXUAL/REPRODUCTIVE ISSUES — When a woman's thyroid hormone levels drop too low, it can affect ovulation, decreasing fertility. The long-term effects of hypothyroidism have also been linked to decreased libido in both men and women.

BIRTH DEFECTS — Untreated hypothyroidism may increase the risk of birth defects such as cleft palate. Children born to women with untreated hypothyroidism are also more likely to experience delays in intellectual and physical development.

MYXEDEMA—When left untreated, hypothyroidism can increase the risk for a rare but life-threatening condition called myxedema. Signs of myxedema include increased sensitivity to cold, drowsiness, and lethargy, often followed eventually by unconsciousness. Because coma is the eventual result of this rare form of hypothyroidism, immediate medical attention is required for patients experiencing extreme fatigue or cold intolerance.

HASHIMOTO'S DISEASE AND PREGNANCY

Hashimoto's disease is more common in women than in men, and pregnant women have a particularly high risk for developing hypothyroidism. According to the National Institutes of Health, hypothyroidism occurs in 3 to 5 out of every 1,000 pregnancies.[18] The thyroid gland plays an important role in pregnancy, both for the health of the mother and for the development of the child.

During pregnancy, the body begins to produce more of certain hormones, namely estrogen and human chorionic gonadotropin (hCG). Produced in the placenta, hCG works in a similar way as TSH, stimulating the thyroid gland to make more thyroid hormone. Increased estrogen levels lead to increased production of thyroid-binding globulin, a type of protein that helps to transport thyroid hormone through the bloodstream. During the first 12 weeks of development, the fetus depends on the mother's supply of thyroid hormones until it is able to regulate thyroid function on its own.[19]

If not controlled during pregnancy, hypothyroidism can lead to preeclampsia, anemia, low birth weight, miscarriage, or stillbirth.

Hashimoto's disease, with or without concurrent hypothyroidism, can be very serious if left untreated. Not only can it lead to complications like hormone imbalance and gut damage, but it can also increase the risk for developing additional autoimmune disorders. Unfortunately, there is no cure for Hashimoto's, but managing the condition through hormone replacement and lifestyle changes can reduce the risk for developing complications. The rest of this book is dedicated to providing you with the information you need to properly manage Hashimoto's. By implementing the dietary and lifestyle changes recommended in this book, you can find relief from Hashimoto's symptoms and go back to living your life.

PART II
TREATING HASHIMOTO'S DISEASE

CHAPTER 3
Methods for Diagnosis

"Blood tests alone cannot always adequately diagnose thyroid hormone imbalance. It is estimated that about forty percent of the U.S. population suffers from some kind of thyroid imbalance as opposed to the current traditional figure of ten percent. This is due to the inadequacies of the TSH test."

—Dr. Nikolas R. Hedberg, *The Thyroid Alternative*[20]

If you are experiencing symptoms of Hashimoto's disease, or if you have some of the previously mentioned risk factors, talk to your physician. Hashimoto's can be tricky to diagnose since the symptoms overlap with a number of other conditions and it often develops without any initial outward signs. Even so, there are several diagnostic tools and tests that your doctor can use to determine whether you have the disease. Once you have a diagnosis, you can begin taking the necessary steps to treat and manage the condition. With proper management, including changes to your diet and lifestyle, it is entirely possible to go into remission. In this chapter you will learn about the various methods used to diagnose Hashimoto's disease.

DIAGNOSING HASHIMOTO'S DISEASE

Diagnosis for any condition begins with a thorough physical exam and a medical history. For many Hashimoto's patients, the first sign is a goiter that forms on the front or side of the neck. During the physical exam, a physician will check for this type of growth as well as the presence of symptoms that are consistent with hypothyroidism. When taking a medical history, the physician will ask about the following:

- Changes in health that may indicate changes in metabolism

- Prior thyroid surgery

- Prior radiation treatment affecting the neck

- Use of medications that may cause hypothyroidism

- A family history of thyroid disease

When the physical exam and medical history point toward a diagnosis of Hashimoto's disease or hypothyroidism, certain blood tests are required in order to confirm the diagnosis. The following are the most common blood tests used to confirm a Hashimoto's diagnosis.

TSH HORMONE TEST — Typically, the first blood test ordered to confirm a diagnosis of Hashimoto's disease is a test for TSH, or thyroid stimulating hormone. As explained in the previous chapter, TSH is a hormone produced by the pituitary gland, which regulates the production and release of thyroid hormone by the thyroid gland. Hypersensitive, the TSH test is able to detect even the slightest amount of thyroid hormone in the blood. It is the most accurate measure of thyroid activity currently available.[21]

In order to confirm thyroid activity, the TSH test must reveal a reading above normal. An above normal reading suggests decreased thyroid activity because the pituitary gland increases TSH production when it senses a decrease in thyroid hormone production. Normal values range from 0.4 to 4.0 milli-international units per liter, or mlU/L. The normal value for this test may vary slightly from one laboratory to another depending on testing methods. A TSH value above 4.0 mlU/L is an indication of hypothyroidism, and it may also support a diagnosis of Hashimoto's disease. If the TSH test reveals a value below normal, it could be an indication of hyperthyroidism, potentially caused by a toxic nodular goiter, Graves' disease, or excessive iodine levels in the body.

T4 TEST—If the TSH test reveals an above-normal reading, a second test called a T4 test might be performed to measure the actual amount of thyroid hormone circulating in the bloodstream. T4 is thyroxine, the main hormone produced by the thyroid gland. To confirm a diagnosis of hypothyroidism, the amount of T4 in the bloodstream must be lower than normal. The normal range for this value is between 4.5 and 11.2 micrograms per deciliter (mcg/dL).

A T4 level that is lower than normal suggests a diagnosis of hypothyroidism, but it could also be an indication of malnutrition or it could be caused by certain medications including anabolic steroids, barbiturates, glucocorticoid medications, and antithyroid drugs. A T4 test that reveals above-normal results could be an indication of Graves' disease, a toxic nodular tumor, trophoblastic disease, subacute thyroiditis, germ cell tumor, or even pregnancy.

T3 TEST—Just as the T4 test measures the amount of thyroxine in your blood, the T3 test measures the amount of triiodothyronine. This test is most commonly administered along with a T4 test to evaluate thyroid function, particularly in cases of hyperthyroidism when T4 levels may be normal but T3 levels could be increased. An above-normal result on a T3 test could indicate Graves' disease, a toxic nodular goiter, or liver disease. Taking certain medications like methadone and birth control pills can increase T3 to above-normal levels.

The normal T3 range is between 100 and 200 nanograms per deciliter (ng/dL). Lower-than-normal results could indicate an underactive thyroid, some kind of illness, or starvation. In most cases, however, abnormally low levels are the result of thyroiditis, the kind of swelling or inflammation of the thyroid gland caused by Hashimoto's disease.

ANTITHYROID ANTIBODY TEST—The final blood test used to confirm a diagnosis of Hashimoto's disease is the antithyroid antibody test. When the body produces an autoimmune response and begins attacking the healthy tissue in the thyroid gland, thyroid autoantibodies are present in the bloodstream. Most people with Hashimoto's disease test positive for these antibodies, and these antibodies are not present in people whose hypothyroidism is caused by a different underlying condition. There are two specific types of antithyroid antibodies that this test can identify:

- Anti-TG antibodies, which attack a specific protein in the thyroid called thyroglobulin.

- Anti-thyroperoxidase (TPO) antibodies, which attack an enzyme in thyroid cells called thyroperoxidase (the enzyme that helps to convert T4 into T3).

While any one of these four blood tests can be used to confirm a diagnosis of hypothyroidism, they may not be enough to confirm a diagnosis of Hashimoto's disease. A positive antithyroid antibody test, of course, is a clear indicator of Hashimoto's, but other tests may still be required to determine the progression of the disease. Two other tests that may be useful in determining the extent of damage caused by Hashimoto's disease are ultrasound and CT scan.

ULTRASOUND — An ultrasound scan creates an image of internal structures within the body. This test works by using a device called a transducer, which bounces sound waves off the internal organs to create the image. A trained technician administers the test, and a doctor specializing in medical imaging analyzes the results. Completely safe and painless, the test can be performed on an outpatient basis, takes only a few minutes, and requires no anesthesia. An ultrasound scan can produce an image of the thyroid gland, showing the size and texture of the gland as well as a pattern of autoimmune inflammation and any nodules or growths that may be present.[22]

CT SCAN — A computerized tomography scan is a type of x-ray that generates cross-sectional views of internal structures. This type of scan is usually administered to determine the placement and size of a goiter, and to show its effect on any nearby structures in the neck. Drinking or being injected with a special dye called a contrast medium before the scan may be necessary to enhance the image.

Each case of Hashimoto's is slightly different, so your doctor may order some of these tests but not others. Using the information gleaned from the test results, your doctor will be able to develop an individualized Hashimoto's treatment plan. In the next chapter you will learn about the various medical treatment options for this condition.

CHAPTER 4
Medical Treatment Options

"Unfortunately, there is no known way to prevent Hashimoto's thyroiditis ... but on the bright side, this disorder is very treatable. The sooner you get diagnosed, the sooner you can start receiving treatment."

—Dr. Kresimira Milas, "Hashimoto's Thyroiditis Overview"[23]

If you have been diagnosed with Hashimoto's disease, you may be wondering if there is anything you could have done to prevent it. While it is possible to prevent hypothyroidism from becoming a serious health problem, there is no sure way to prevent the condition from developing if you have the risk factor—this is especially true for hypothyroidism caused by Hashimoto's disease. Hashimoto's is the result of a malfunction in the immune system, and that is not something you can control.

Although it is impossible to prevent Hashimoto's disease or concurrent hypothyroidism, a number of treatment options are available. The treatment plan for Hashimoto's will vary from one individual to another, largely dependent on the extent of thyroid damage at the point of diagnosis. If the condition hasn't progressed to full-blown hypothyroidism, there may be options available to treat the symptoms and improve thyroid function. Once hypothyroidism comes into effect, however, it becomes necessary to supplement the body's natural production of thyroid hormone with replacement thyroid hormone. Additional therapies with iodine supplementation, and changes to diet and lifestyle may also be beneficial.

THYROID HORMONE REPLACEMENT THERAPY

When the body can no longer produce thyroid hormone, or if it is unable to produce enough, thyroid hormone replacement therapy is necessary. This is the most common medical treatment for hypothyroidism and Hashimoto's disease. To understand how this type of hormone replacement therapy works, you must first understand the interaction between the two thyroid hormones, T3 and T4.

T3 is the more active of the two thyroid hormones. T4 is sometimes called a prohormone because the body can convert it into T3. When T4 interacts with other cells in the bloodstream, it loses an iodine atom during the interaction, which converts it into T3. Although both of these hormones are necessary, T3 is the stronger of the two because it is derived from T4. Together, T3 and T4 regulate metabolic rate, which determines the rate at which the body processes food, the speed at which the heart beats, and the body's ability to regulate body temperature.

Because T3 is stronger, you might expect thyroid hormone replacement therapy to consist of taking synthetic T3. In reality, most hormone replacement therapy for hypothyroidism involves taking synthetic T4. This is the case for two reasons. One reason is that supplementing your body's supply of T4 hormone allows it to maintain normal metabolic function in converting T4 into T3. The other reason is that T4 has a longer half-life than T3 (7 days compared with 24 hours), so it will remain in circulation in your body longer.[24]

When it comes to thyroid hormone replacement therapy, there is no cookie-cutter treatment plan. The purpose of treatment is to supplement your body's natural production of thyroid hormone, so the amount of supplementary hormone required depends on the amount of natural hormone your body is still producing. It is also important to realize that each person's body responds differently to the hormone, and it will take some experimentation to find the right dosage in response to your body's absorption and utilization of the hormone.

Not only will dosage amounts vary, but there are also different types of supplementary hormone that may be prescribed. Synthetic T4, typically in pill form, is most commonly prescribed. An animal thyroid supplement may be prescribed in certain cases. Synthetic T3 is typically reserved for people who have undergone thyroid surgery or prior to the administration of treatments for thyroid cancer.

The most commonly used form of synthetic T4 is levothyroxine sodium, though there are many different brand names for this drug, including Levoxyl, Levo-T, Synthroid, Unithroid, Thyrolar, Levothyroid, and Tirosint. Each of these brand-name medications is bioequivalent, meaning there are no significant differences in biological composition. This does not mean that all are the same in terms of bioavailability and dosage. For example, Synthroid is the most commonly prescribed brand because it offers a steady, prolonged dose of synthetic T4 hormone. Different brands may work better for different patients. Whether you take a brand name drug or a generic version, however, the American Association of Clinical Endocrinologists recommends that you stick with a particular formula once you start treatments, although adjustments can be made to dosage as needed.[25]

Finding the right dosage for synthetic T4 treatments can be tricky because the hormones affect each person differently, and using the wrong dosage can be very dangerous. The correct dosage will keep hypothyroidism at bay, enabling the body to resume normal or near-normal function. The incorrect dosage could exacerbate thyroid issues. In most cases, doctors calculate dosage according to weight, using about 1.6 micrograms per kilogram (2.2 pounds) of bodyweight. Adjustments can be made after a few weeks of hormone replacement therapy, once its effects can be measured.

If you are taking or thinking about taking synthetic T4 hormone, it is imperative that you follow your doctor's advice and be very careful about maintaining the proper dosage. It is easy to overdose on synthetic T4. Negative side effects including the following:

- Sweating more than normal

- Heart palpitations

- Shaking, trembling hands

- Difficulty falling asleep

- Mood swings and irritability

- Mental fog

- Muscle weakness

- Unexplained weight loss

- Menstrual irregularities

If you maintain the proper dosage and take the hormone consistently, you should start to feel the effects within about 2 weeks. If you find that synthetic hormone does not work for you, or if you simply want to learn about your options, there is an alternative to synthetic T4 available: animal thyroid hormone.

The most popular brand of animal thyroid hormone is Armour, a combination of T3 and T4 made from desiccated pig thyroid glands. Animal hormone was the standard throughout the 1800s and well into the 1900s until synthetic thyroid hormone began to take rise.

While animal thyroid hormones are more "natural" than synthetic hormone, there are some factors to consider before deciding on this treatment. For example, just because the treatment is natural doesn't mean that it is safe. First, animal thyroid hormone cannot be purified the way synthetic hormone can, and it is difficult to judge the effects of impure hormone on the body. Second, the actual amount of T3 and T4 in the animal thyroid pills is much less precise than the amount of T4 in synthetic hormone and may vary from one brand to another. Finally, it is important to note that hormone balance in the body of an animal is much different than in the human body, so it is difficult to say for sure that animal thyroid hormone is an effective treatment for humans.[26]

VITAMIN AND MINERAL SUPPLEMENTS

Because multivitamins can contain supplements that may interfere with your Hashimoto's medication, you may want to consider taking individual vitamin and mineral supplements that will benefit your body instead. Here are some of the vitamins and minerals that will benefit patients struggling with Hashimoto's disease.

ZINC — People with Hashimoto's disease and/or hypothyroidism often have a zinc deficiency. Zinc plays a key role in supporting healthy immune function, and it is a powerful anti-inflammatory as well, helping to reduce oxidative stress and chronic inflammation.

Additionally, zinc helps to control the body's immune response, which could help to reduce autoimmunity — this is particularly beneficial for Hashimoto's disease.[27] There is a delicate balance between adequate zinc levels and overdose, so be very careful when taking zinc supplements.[28]

SELENIUM — This mineral plays an important role in the conversion of T4 to T3. It is possible to have normal levels of T4 in your bloodstream even if you are deficient in selenium and zinc, but your body will not be able to complete the conversion process normally. As an anti-inflammatory agent, selenium can help to reduce autoimmunity and slow the progression of Hashimoto's disease. You can take oral selenium supplements on a daily basis or drink a cup of coconut milk beverage to get your daily recommended value.[29]

IODINE — One of the most important supplements for healthy thyroid function is iodine. Unfortunately, people with Hashimoto's or hypothyroidism can develop an increased sensitivity to iodine, potentially to the point where eating iodine-rich foods or taking iodine drops can worsen hypothyroid symptoms. Consult your doctor to determine your daily recommended value for iodine, which will vary depending on a number of factors such as age, sex, and weight. Pregnant women have an increased need for iodine to help support the growth and development of the fetus.

MAGNESIUM — Many people with Hashimoto's disease and hypothyroidism are deficient in magnesium. This mineral plays an important role in helping the body absorb and utilize iodine — this is why iodine deficiencies and magnesium deficiencies frequently occur together. You can increase your consumption of avocados, fish, and dark leafy greens to boost your daily magnesium intake. While magnesium can be beneficial for Hashimoto's patients it can also interfere with Hashimoto's medications if taken within 4 hours of T4 treatment. If you are taking both magnesium supplements and T4 treatments, be sure to space them at least 4 hours apart.

B VITAMINS — These vitamins play a role in supporting optimal thyroid health. Much like magnesium, B vitamins help the body absorb and utilize iodine at the cellular level. Vitamins B2 and B6 are particularly valuable for immune system support.

VITAMIN D — This vitamin plays a key role in maintaining a healthy immune system, so it can be a very beneficial supplement for people with an autoimmune disease like Hashimoto's. Support for this theory comes from a number of studies that showed people suffering from tuberculosis responded well to natural sunlight and many patients suffering from this disease also experience autoimmune disease. The effects of supplemental vitamin D on immunity are still being studied.[30]

ADDITIONAL SUPPLEMENTS

DSF — A type of adrenal support supplement, DSF supplements can be very useful for people with Hashimoto's or hypothyroidism. As previously mentioned, adrenal function is closely linked to thyroid function so taking a supplement like this could help your body recover from thyroid damage. This supplement contains vitamins, minerals, antioxidants, glandulars (animal tissues which can neutralize antigen-antibody reactions), and phytochemicals (chemical compounds found in plants which can reduce the risk for chronic disease), all of which work together to keep the body functioning properly.[31]

FISH OIL — Essential fatty acids (both omega-3s and omega-6s) play a key role in reducing inflammation. Chronic inflammation is a common side effect of autoimmune disease, so taking fish oil supplements on a daily basis may help to keep this particular side effect under control. In general, fatty acids have also been known to help enhance T-cell (a type of white blood cell) function.

ECHINACEA — You may already be familiar with echinacea as a natural supplement for preventing or reducing the severity of colds. Its immune-boosting effects could potentially be beneficial for sufferers of autoimmune conditions, although there is no definitive evidence yet to confirm this theory.[32]

PROBIOTICS — Because 80 percent of the immune system is located in the gut, many autoimmune conditions like Hashimoto's contribute to gut imbalances or leaky gut syndrome (see page 222) for more on these conditions. Taking a daily probiotic helps to restore the natural flora in the digestive tract, improving digestive function and reducing autoimmunity.[33]

SUPPLEMENTS THAT MAY INTERFERE WITH HASHIMOTO'S TREATMENT

In addition to thyroid hormone replacement therapy, other supplements may be prescribed to help manage your Hashimoto's or hypothyroid symptoms. It is important to note that certain medications and supplements can actually interfere with your body's ability to absorb and utilize the synthetic hormone, so follow your doctor's instructions very carefully and check for any drug interactions on the pharmacy label. Medications or supplements that may interfere with synthetic T4 if taken within 4 hours of treatment include:

- Calcium supplements

- Aluminum hydroxide (found in antacids)

- Iron supplements

- Colestid and cholestyramine (drugs to reduce cholesterol)

- Magnesium supplements

- Sucralfate (ulcer treatment)

- Raloxifene (osteoporosis treatment)

- Soy-based foods

If you do need to take any of these medications or supplements, you can still do so even if you are on a synthetic hormone medication—just be aware that these supplements may affect your body's ability to absorb the synthetic hormone. The best way to avoid negative interactions between your Hashimoto's thyroid medication and any supplements you are taking is to wait 4 hours after taking your thyroid hormone to take any additional supplements. In many cases, it is recommended that you take the thyroid pill either first thing in the morning or at night before bed, so it should be easy to work in your other supplements around this schedule.

Although some supplements have the potential to interfere with Hashimoto's medication, certain supplements can be very beneficial if taken concurrently with thyroid hormone replacement therapy.

By now you should have a basic understanding of the various treatments available for Hashimoto's disease as well as how each of the treatments works. It is up to you and your doctor to create a customized treatment plan and, once you do, it is imperative that you stick to it. Once you start hormone replacement therapy you should start to feel the effects of the treatment within 2 weeks or so. Be sure to keep routine follow-up appointments with your physician, and take note of any side effects you may experience.

CHAPTER 5
Dietary Recommendations

"The Autoimmune Protocol (AIP) [is] a Paleo-style diet that provides nutritious foods while promoting gut healing and reducing inflammation ... The Paleo diet takes a simple approach to food. It is an eating lifestyle based on that of our human ancestors. People on the Paleo diet eat foods that most closely approximate what our ancestors ate: seasonal whole foods that can be hunted or gathered."

—Karen Frazier, *The Hashimoto's Cookbook and Action Plan*[34]

While the primary course of treatment for Hashimoto's disease is thyroid hormone replacement therapy, there are also dietary and lifestyle changes you can make to supplement your medical treatment. Certain dietary and lifestyle habits have been linked to autoimmune disease and to Hashimoto's disease in particular, so making an effort to break those habits could help to ensure the success of your treatment plan. Remember, Hashimoto's affects each person differently so the dietary changes that might work to reduce Hashimoto's symptoms in one person may not be effective in another person. In the same way that you may need to tweak the dosage of your synthetic hormone treatment, you may need to experiment with different dietary modifications so the diet works for you.

In this chapter you will learn the basics about dietary recommendations for Hashimoto's patients. You will discover which foods can trigger or exacerbate immune response as well as which foods are beneficial for your immune system and your thyroid gland. You will also find dietary recommendations for how many servings to consume from each of the main food groups each day. A number of diets have been designed to help treat autoimmune disease or thyroid problems, and the recommendations in this chapter combine the key elements from each of those diets to help you maximize your healing potential.

GOALS OF DIETARY CHANGES FOR HASHIMOTO'S

The goals of the Hashimoto's diet are to reduce chronic inflammation, balance hormones, and repair autoimmune damage (particularly gut damage). Although each person responds to Hashimoto's and hypothyroidism in a different way, certain dietary changes are known to be beneficial for autoimmune and thyroid conditions generally. These are the recommended dietary changes that will help you to achieve the above goals. You may have to tweak your diet here and there, but the best way to start building a Hashimoto's diet is on a gluten-free, Paleo foundation.

BASIC DIETARY RECOMMENDATIONS

The Hashimoto's diet is a Paleo and gluten-free diet designed to repair the damage caused by your body's own autoimmune response. Autoimmune diseases like Hashimoto's respond very well to elimination diets like the Paleo diet. An elimination diet requires you to remove certain foods or types of foods from your diet and, in doing so, give your body a chance to heal and recover from autoimmune damage. After the recovery period you may choose to reintroduce potentially problematic foods one at a time to gauge your body's response. If you experience a negative reaction, you should continue to omit those foods from your diet. Though elimination diets like the Paleo diet are highly effective for autoimmune disease, it is important to remember that Hashimoto's is more than just an autoimmune disease—it is also a thyroid condition, so additional dietary modifications are required to restore thyroid function.

THE PALEO AUTOIMMUNE PROTOCOL

Hashimoto's diet plan is based on the Paleo Autoimmune Protocol (AIP), which is a Paleo, gluten-free diet designed to alleviate symptoms caused by autoimmune disease. Although released only recently, AIP is a dietary approach many years in the making. It began with a paper, coauthored by radiologist S. Boyd Eaton. This paper, titled "Paleolithic Nutrition," was published in 1985 in the *New England Journal of Medicine*. The paper explored the potential health benefits of following a Paleolithic-style nutrition plan and has influenced the work and studies of many physicians and researchers, especially in the treatment of autoimmune disease. Loren Cordain, an exercise physiologist specializing in nutrition, is generally credited with doing much of the research that led to the creation of the AIP protocol, but the first book written entirely about the protocol was *The Paleo Approach*. This book was written by Sarah Ballantyne, a scientist and medical researcher, and was published in 2013.

The AIP is not just a fad diet—it is designed to be a long-term lifestyle change to help you reduce and control your Hashimoto's symptoms. By combining this diet with your medical therapies, you may even be able to reverse your hypothyroidism and put your Hashimoto's into remission.[35]

AIP is based on the Paleo diet, which focuses on fresh, whole foods that have been minimally processed or otherwise affected by humans. The common misconception is that the Paleo diet is all about meat (especially bacon), but that is an oversimplification. The true heart of the Paleo diet is wholesome foods that are naturally loaded with nutrients. This includes foods like fresh fruits and vegetables, lean meats and seafood, raw nuts and seeds, healthy fats and oils, and fresh herbs and spices.

Whole foods, like those included in the Paleo diet, are rich in a number of beneficial compounds that help the body heal from chronic inflammation and other impacts of Hashimoto's disease. For example, whole plant foods are rich in phytonutrients, which have natural disease-preventive properties. Phytonutrients (also known as phytochemicals) include antioxidants, which protect cells against free-radical damage; flavonoids, which have anti-inflammatory benefits; and polyphenols, which can reduce the effects of oxidative stress, one of the primary causes for chronic diseases like heart disease, type 2 diabetes, and cancer. Whole foods are also rich in essential vitamins and minerals, in addition to being healthy sources of the three key macronutrients: proteins, carbohydrates, and fats.[36]

The Paleo diet leaves out any foods that weren't readily available to our Paleolithic ancestors. During the Paleolithic era, humans were hunter-gatherers; they subsisted on food that could be caught or gathered. This includes fresh meats and fish, fruits and vegetables, nuts, and seeds. The modern Paleo diet starts with this foundation, but it has been expanded to incorporate other staples such as natural sweeteners, healthy oils, fresh and dried herbs, and spices. Basically, the Paleo diet includes any food that has been minimally altered by humans or does not require pasteurization or processing to make it edible.

THE MAIN FOOD GROUPS OF THE HASHIMOTO'S DIET

The AIP starts with the Paleo diet as a foundation because it includes foods that are naturally nutrient-dense and unlikely to contribute to leaky gut or other intestinal problems. The wholesome, natural foods on which the AIP is founded are also known to reduce inflammation, regulate hormonal balance, and reduce micronutrient deficiencies. The Hashimoto's diet is largely based on the AIP, but it diverges in a number of important ways, particularly in the foods and food groups to avoid because of their potential to contribute to autoimmune disease and hypothyroid problems. For example, the Hashimoto's diet is focused on fresh fruits and vegetables, lean meats and seafood, healthy fats, coconut products, and fermented foods. Additional thyroid-healing foods that are rich in iodine, selenium, and other key nutrients are also important. For the most part, these foods align with the AIP. In terms of foods that are excluded from the diet, the AIP excludes beans and legumes, gluten, grains, dairy products, soy products, sugar, and artificial sweeteners. Where the Hashimoto's diet diverges from the AIP is in the additional exclusions of goitrogenic foods, nuts, seeds, eggs, and nightshade vegetables. These food groups are explained in detail below.

VEGETABLES — Raw and home-cooked vegetables are loaded with healthy nutrients that can boost overall nutrition and help to heal the digestive system. Starchy vegetables like pumpkin, squash, and (in moderation) sweet potato can help to meet the body's needs for complex carbohydrates in addition to increasing the intake of dietary fiber. Complex carbohydrates provide the body with slow-burning energy and dietary fiber essential for healthy digestion. With the exception of starchy or root vegetables, nightshades (page 53), and goitrogenic vegetables (page 49), you can enjoy all other vegetables freely.

FRUITS — Fresh and frozen fruits are rich in dietary fiber and healthy nutrients, and they can help to satisfy your sweet tooth without refined or artificial sugars. Many fruits like blueberries, oranges, and cherries are also rich in antioxidants, which help to heal cells from free-radical damage. Just be sure to limit consumption of goitrogenic fruits like strawberries, peaches, and pears. Enjoy dried fruits in moderation because they have more concentrated fructose than a similar-sized serving of fresh fruit — you should also ensure that any dried or frozen fruits you enjoy have no added sugar; aim to limit your daily sugar consumption to no more than 20 grams daily. This equates to about 2 medium apples, 2 cups of grapes, 5 cups of berries, or 1 cup of dried fruit.

LEAN MEATS AND SEAFOOD — The best protein sources for the Hashimoto's diet are lean cuts of grass-fed meats, free-range poultry, and wild-caught fish and seafood.

HEALTHY FATS — The best healthy fats and oils to use on the Hashimoto's diet include avocado, coconut oil, grass-fed ghee, lard, extra virgin olive oil, palm oil, and tallow. Animal fats like lard and tallow are rich in flavor as well as omega-3 fatty acids — omega-3 fatty acids support healthy thyroid function and may also help to improve hormone balance. The fats and oils listed here are rich in monounsaturated fats and medium-chain triglycerides (MCTs), both of which help to reduce inflammation and boost immunity. Ghee is clarified butter from which milk proteins and sugars (like lactose and casein) have been removed. It is regarded as a Paleo-friendly fat by many, but you should see how your body responds to it.

HERBS AND SPICES — Fresh and dried herbs and spices are not only rich in nutrients, but they are a great way to add flavor to foods. Enjoy basil, cilantro, parsley, dill, and other leafy herbs as well as garlic, a bulb, and ginger, a rhizome. Be sure to avoid herbs and spices that come from seeds (such as cumin, coriander, and nutmeg) as well as peppers such as cayenne, chili powder, and paprika.

COCONUT PRODUCTS — Fresh coconut and coconut products like coconut milk, coconut flour, and coconut oil are loaded with nutrients that are good for the immune system. Coconut contains nutrients and compounds with natural antiviral, antibacterial, and antifungal properties, not to mention plenty of healthy fat.

FERMENTED FOODS — One of the major goals of the Hashimoto's diet is to heal the digestive system, and fermented foods are a powerful tool for digestion. The process of fermenting significantly increases digestive enzymes in a food, making it a natural probiotic.[37] Some examples of fermented foods and beverages to enjoy on the Hashimoto's diet are coconut yogurt, kombucha, water kefir, and fermented vegetables — as long as they are not nightshades (page 53) or goitrogenic foods (page 49).

ADDITIONAL FOODS — Vinegars such as balsamic vinegar, cider vinegar, red wine vinegar, and white wine vinegar are allowed on the Hashimoto's diet. Small amounts of natural sweeteners such as honey and pure maple syrup are also permitted. As for beverages, focus on herbal teas, green tea, and water — and avoid alcohol and sugary beverages.

THYROID-HEALING FOODS

In addition to increasing your consumption of the various foods listed above, try to eat more of the following mineral-rich foods, which may help to heal your thyroid.

IODINE-RICH FOODS—Foods high in iodine may help to reverse thyroid damage. Some examples are iodized salt and sea vegetables like kelp, kombu, nori, and wakame, as well as lesser sources like cranberries, cod, shrimp, bananas, and green beans.

SELENIUM-RICH FOODS—Foods rich in selenium include seafood, shellfish, poultry, pork, and red meats.

FOODS HIGH IN ZINC, MAGNESIUM, AND VITAMINS B AND D—These vitamins and minerals are thyroid boosters. Foods rich in zinc include lean beef and poultry, oysters, and crab. Food sources of magnesium include leafy greens, avocados, bananas, and fish. B vitamins are found in most animal products. Beef liver, orange juice, mushrooms, and fatty fish are among the foods rich in vitamin D.

Depending on your treatment plan, your physician may recommend that you take dietary supplements to increase your daily intake. Keep in mind that natural sources of vitamins and minerals are much more valuable because your body can digest and absorb them more efficiently. However, if you are having trouble meeting your daily intake with natural sources, dietary supplements are a good alternative.

FOODS TO AVOID

The Paleo diet calls for avoiding grains and legumes because they have been altered by humans and are produced through agricultural practices not available during the Paleolithic era. Processed sugar and alcohol products are also excluded from the diet, as are dairy products since they too come from the agricultural practice of raising livestock. In short, the Paleo diet is a gluten-free, grain-free, sugar-free (except for natural sweeteners), and dairy-free diet.[38] This is the foundation on which the Autoimmune Protocol is built, but the Hashimoto's diet calls for some additional exclusions such as goitrogenic foods, nuts, seeds, eggs, and nightshade vegetables.

GOITROGENIC FOODS

Many people who have iodine deficiency–induced hypo-thyroidism find that consuming goitrogenic foods exacerbates their Hashimoto's symptoms. These foods contain compounds called goitrogens which can impair the ability of the thyroid to produce thyroid hormones. Goitrogenic foods can affect the thyroid in different ways, and certain goitrogenic foods have a greater effect on the thyroid than others. For example, cruciferous vegetables may inhibit iodine metabolism, which can impact healthy thyroid function, and they may induce the production of antibodies that may cross-react with the thyroid gland.[39]

There is a great deal of controversy in the medical community about the potentially harmful effects of goitrogenic foods—while some of these foods simply do not agree with certain people, many of them contain valuable nutrients and other beneficial compounds that can actually support healthy thyroid function. For example, goitrogenous cruciferous vegetables, like broccoli and cauliflower, are rich in cancer-fighting antioxidants while goitrogenous root vegetables, like sweet potatoes and turnips, are healthy sources of complex carbohydrates. Strawberries and sweet potatoes are rich in carotenoids, while other fruits and vegetables contain an assortment of essential vitamins and minerals.

When it comes to consuming goitrogenic foods on the Hashimoto's diet, it is best to limit your consumption for the first 30 days until your body heals from the thyroid damage. After this point you may choose to reintroduce these foods slowly, as long as your body is able to tolerate them. While limiting your consumption of goitrogenic foods for the first 30 days, it is best to consume no more than 6 to 8 servings of goitrogenic fruits and vegetables per week. You can deactivate the goitrogenic activity of these foods and further minimize any potential negative effects by cooking, steaming, or fermenting them, though eating raw goitrogenic foods in 2 to 3 servings per week is generally not harmful. One serving of goitrogenic food is equal to 2 cups of raw leafy greens, 1 cup of cooked fruits or vegetables, or ½ cup of raw fruits or vegetables.

Goitrogenic foods are:

- Gluten-containing foods

- Soy products such as edamame, tempeh, tofu

- Canola

- Cruciferous vegetables such as arugula, bok choy, broccoli, broccoli rabe, brussels sprouts, cabbage, cauliflower, Chinese (Napa) cabbage, collard greens, kale, kohlrabi, mustard greens, turnip greens, watercress

- Certain root vegetables such as cassava, horseradish, rutabaga, sweet potato, turnips, wasabi

- Certain fruits such as peaches, pears, strawberries

- Spinach

- Certain nuts, seeds, and legumes (flaxseed, pine nuts, peanuts)

GLUTEN — Not only are gluten-containing foods potential goitrogens, but they commonly pose a problem for individuals with autoimmune disease. A type of protein found in wheat, barley, rye, and triticale, gluten is found in many processed foods and convenience foods. Removing gluten from the diet can help to reduce inflammation (particularly in the gut), and it may help to reduce psychological and mental problems such as depression, irritability, brain fog, and memory issues.

GRAINS — The Paleo diet calls for avoiding all grains — including oats, corn, quinoa, rice, and millet — and not just gluten-containing grains. Consumption of grains has been linked to chronic inflammation, and it may also exacerbate the symptoms of autoimmune disease in some people. For individuals with Hashimoto's disease, eating grains can contribute to blood sugar imbalance, which can affect hormone levels, and hormone balance is essential in managing Hashimoto's. After 30 days or so on the diet, you may be able to reintroduce non-gluten grains one at a time to see which ones, if any, your body tolerates.

LEGUMES — This food group includes beans, chickpeas, lentils, peas, and peanuts. Legumes contain phytates as well as lectins, a compound also found in grains, which can spark autoimmune reactions in some people. Legumes have also been linked to chronic inflammation and leaky gut syndrome so they should be avoided on the Hashimoto's diet. Fresh green beans are considered safe because they contain much less of the harmful compounds such as phytates and lectins which are found in dried beans and legumes. In large quantities, these compounds can damage the lining of your intestines and interfere with nutrient absorption.

DAIRY — Milk and milk products contain two substances that can be harmful to people with autoimmune and thyroid problems: casein and lactose. Casein, a protein, is very similar in biological structure to gluten. Lactose is a type of sugar that many people have trouble digesting. As with non-gluten grains, you may be able to reintroduce dairy products one at a time to see if your body can handle them. Wait until you've been on the diet 30 days or so before trying it.

SUGAR AND ARTIFICIAL SWEETENERS — Eating too much sugar can raise blood sugar and insulin levels as well as increase inflammation in the body. Avoid all forms of processed sugar including brown sugar, high-fructose corn syrup, molasses, powdered sugar, and white sugar. Also avoid artificial sweeteners such as aspartame, sucralose, and sugar alcohols. You may, however, enjoy small amounts of natural sweeteners — raw honey, agave, and pure maple syrup — but no more than 1 tablespoon per day.

UNHEALTHY FATS — Avoid all trans fats, vegetables oils and vegetable shortening. Trans fats are produced by hydrogenating vegetable oils and they can increase your LDL or "bad cholesterol" levels while reducing your HDL or "good cholesterol" levels. You should also avoid nut oils and seed oils such as almond oil and sesame oil. Healthy oils like coconut oil, olive oil, and palm oil are permitted.

SOY PRODUCTS — Anyone with any type of autoimmune disease should avoid soy products, including tofu, bean sprouts, edamame, miso, MSG, soy sauce, tempeh, teriyaki sauce, and textured vegetable protein. In the United States, more than 90 percent of soy crops have been genetically modified — genetically modified crops often contain high levels of chemical pesticides and insecticides, toxins which can trigger autoimmune disease. Additionally, soy is a legume and a highly goitrogenic food so it should be excluded from the Hashimoto's diet.

NUTS AND SEEDS — While nuts and seeds are allowed on the Paleo diet, they are not included in the AIP or the Hashimoto's diet. Tree nuts are among the most common causes of food allergies, and both nuts and seeds have been known to cause problems for individuals with autoimmune disease. Avoid all nuts and seeds including butters, flours, and oils made from either nuts or seeds.

EGGS — Another common allergenic food, eggs have been known to cause problems for people with autoimmune disease. They may also contribute to gut inflammation and leaky gut syndrome. Egg whites are particularly problematic, although you should avoid both whites and yolks for at least 30 days while following the Hashimoto's diet. After this time you may be able to reintroduce eggs once your body has healed from chronic inflammation and gut damage.

NIGHTSHADES — This family of plants is known to cause inflammation and may also contribute to leaky gut syndrome and autoimmune disease because they can cause inflammation and reduce the body's ability to absorb key nutrients like vitamin D. Nightshades include tomatoes, potatoes, eggplant, peppers, and tomatillos as well as certain spices like paprika, cayenne, and chili powder.

DIETARY MISTAKES TO AVOID

Crafting a diet to minimize Hashimoto's disease and hypothyroid symptoms can be tricky, especially since each person's body reacts differently to dietary changes. Here are a few dietary mistakes that everyone with Hashimoto's disease should avoid.

FOODS TO ENJOY FREELY		FOODS TO ENJOY IN MODERATION
VEGETABLES ▪ artichoke ▪ asparagus ▪ beet greens ▪ celery ▪ cucumber ▪ endive ▪ green beans ▪ jicama ▪ lettuce ▪ mushrooms ▪ okra ▪ onion ▪ summer squash FRUIT ▪ apple ▪ apricot ▪ banana ▪ blackberries ▪ blueberries ▪ cherries ▪ cranberries ▪ dates ▪ fig ▪ grapefruit ▪ grapes ▪ kiwi ▪ lemon ▪ lime ▪ melon ▪ mango ▪ orange ▪ papaya ▪ pineapple ▪ plum ▪ pomegranate ▪ raspberries ▪ watermelon HERBS ▪ basil ▪ cilantro ▪ cinnamon ▪ garlic ▪ ginger	▪ mint ▪ oregano ▪ parsley ▪ thyme FERMENTED FOODS ▪ coconut yogurt ▪ fermented vegetables ▪ kombucha ▪ vinegar ▪ water kefir HEALTHY FATS ▪ avocado oil ▪ coconut oil ▪ grass-fed ghee ▪ lard ▪ olive oil ▪ palm oil MEAT *(grass-fed)* ▪ beef ▪ lamb ▪ veal ▪ pork ▪ venison ▪ bison POULTRY *(free-range)* ▪ chicken ▪ turkey ▪ quail ▪ pheasant ▪ duck SEAFOOD *(wild-caught)* ▪ fish ▪ shellfish OTHER ▪ bone broth ▪ coconut products (oil, aminos, cream, milk, unsweetened shredded coconut) ▪ tea (black, green, and herbal)	GOITROGENIC VEGETABLES ▪ arugula ▪ bok choy ▪ broccoli ▪ brussels sprouts ▪ cabbage ▪ cassava ▪ cauliflower ▪ collard greens ▪ horseradish ▪ kale ▪ kohlrabi ▪ mustard greens ▪ radish ▪ rutabaga ▪ sweet potato ▪ turnips ▪ watercress OTHER VEGETABLES ▪ beet root ▪ butternut squash ▪ carrot ▪ pumpkin ▪ parsnip ▪ spinach ▪ squash GOITROGENIC FRUIT ▪ peaches ▪ pears ▪ strawberries NATURAL SWEETENERS ▪ agave ▪ pure maple syrup ▪ raw honey

FOODS TO AVOID COMPLETELY
AVOID ALL NIGHTSHADES AND SEEDS, INCLUDING THE FOLLOWING:

VEGETABLES
- eggplant
- peppers
- potatoes
- tomatillos
- tomatoes

HERBS
- caraway
- cardamom
- cayenne pepper
- chili powder
- coriander
- cumin
- dill (seed only)
- fennel
- fenugreek
- mustard seed
- nutmeg
- paprika

BEANS/LEGUMES
- black beans
- chickpeas
- kidney beans
- lentils
- navy beans
- peanuts
- peas
- pinto beans
- soy products
- split peas
- white beans

DAIRY
- butter
- buttermilk
- cheese
- condensed milk
- cottage cheese
- cream
- cream cheese
- custard
- evaporated milk
- frozen yogurt
- ice cream
- milk
- sour cream
- yogurt

EGGS (*at least 30 days*)

UNHEALTHY FATS
- canola oil
- corn oil
- hydrogenated oil
- peanut oil
- rapeseed oil
- safflower oil
- soybean oil
- transfats

NON-GLUTENOUS GRAINS (*at least 30 days*)
- amaranth
- buckwheat
- corn
- couscous
- Kamut
- millet
- oats
- quinoa
- rice
- sorghum
- spelt
- teff

GLUTENOUS GRAINS
- barley
- rye
- triticale
- wheat

NUTS
- almonds
- brazil nuts
- cashews
- chestnuts
- hazelnuts
- macadamia nuts
- pecans
- pine nuts
- pistachios
- walnuts
- nut oils, flours, and butters

SEEDS
- chia
- flax
- hemp
- poppy
- pumpkin
- sesame
- sunflower
- seed oils, flours, and butters

SOY PRODUCTS
- edamame
- tempeh
- tofu

SUGAR AND ARTIFICIAL SWEETENERS
- brown sugar
- corn sugar
- corn syrup
- cane sugar
- high fructose malt syrup
- molasses
- powdered sugar
- white sugar
- aspartame
- mannitol
- stevia
- sucralose
- sugar alcohols
- xylitol

OTHER
- alcohol
- chocolate
- coffee (*at least 30 days*)
- processed foods

RESTRICTED-CALORIE DIETS—Calorie restriction can actually worsen thyroid problems. When you reduce your calorie consumption too severely, your body goes into starvation mode and increases production of reverse T3, inactive form of the T3 hormone, to preserve energy. As a result, thyroid hormone production slows down and total thyroid function could decrease by as much as 50 percent after a few weeks of calorie restriction.[40]

LOW-FAT DIETS—Often, low-fat diets are high in sugar. Why is this the case? In creating low-fat versions of packaged foods, manufacturers alter the oils they use to produce the foods. Because this alteration changes the taste and texture of those foods, the manufacturers increase the sugar content to make the foods palatable.[41] This may be the reason why so many people struggle to lose weight after they start eating diet foods. The foods also contribute to an increased risk for insulin resistance and related hormone imbalances—and elevated insulin levels in the blood (and insulin resistance) can contribute to thyroid resistance and the increased production of reverse T3.

LOW-CARB DIETS—Carbohydrates provide the body with instant fuel that can be converted into the energy needed to carry out metabolic tasks. When you consume carbohydrates, your body produces insulin to help break the food down into glucose and then convert the glucose into energy. When you decrease your carbohydrate consumption, you also decrease your insulin levels. Insulin is very important for healthy thyroid function; it aids the conversion of inactive T4 into active T3. Low-carb diets can also lead to a condition known as "adrenal fatigue" and, as mentioned earlier, adrenal function is closely related to thyroid function.[42]

THE DETAILS OF THE HASHIMOTO'S DIET

Now that you understand a little more about how certain foods and food groups can negatively impact your body, you are ready to learn the basics of the Hashimoto's diet. Again, this diet is based on the foundational principles of the Autoimmune Protocol with a few modifications to help reduce inflammation, restore gut health, and balance hormones.

SERVING SIZES AND RECOMMENDATIONS

How much should you eat from each food group? (See page 45 for the breakdown of food groups.) The best advice is to follow a moderate protein, moderate carbohydrate, and moderate fat diet. Basically, you should build a diet that is as evenly balanced as possible to ensure that your body gets the nutrients it needs in the right ratios. Aim for a moderate carbohydrate consumption around 20 to 30 percent of your daily calories, keeping in mind that your daily carbs should come from gluten-free and grain-free sources like squash and root vegetables. Plan to consume about 20 grams of protein at each meal from approved sources, and don't be afraid to consume healthy fats and oils. You can use free mobile or online applications like My Fitness Pal to track your macronutrient ratios. Limit your consumption of natural sweeteners as well as fruit. Here is a summary of daily dietary recommendations for the Hashimoto's diet.

TYPE OF FOOD	SERVING SIZE EXAMPLE	DAILY SERVINGS	FOODS TO AVOID/LIMIT
Protein (grass-fed meat, poultry, and seafood)	3 ounces cooked (about the size of your palm)	3	None
Raw or cooked vegetables	2 cups raw leafy greens OR 1 cup raw or cooked vegetables	4–5	Avoid nightshades Limit goitrogenic vegetables and fruits to 6–8 total servings per week
Fruit	1 medium apple OR 1 cup fresh berries OR ¼ cup (1 ounce) dried fruit	2	Limit goitrogenic vegetables and fruits to 6–8 total servings per week
Healthy fats and oils	1 tablespoon	4–6	None
Starchy and root vegetables (complex carbohydrates)	1 cup cooked winter squash	1–2	Limit goitrogenic vegetables and fruits to 6–8 total servings per week
Natural sweetener	1 tablespoon honey, agave, or maple syrup	1	None

To help you understand what foods you should eat or avoid on the Hashimoto's diet, consult the food lists on page 54.

TIPS FOR VEGANS AND VEGETARIANS

The Hashimoto's diet includes animal products such as grass-fed meats, poultry, and seafood, but it is possible to follow the diet if you are vegan or vegetarian. Of course, the challenge with any vegan or vegetarian diet is getting enough protein. Many vegans and vegetarians obtain their daily protein from high-protein soy, beans, legumes, nuts, seeds, and grains, but none of these foods are allowed on the Hashimoto's diet plan. Add to this challenge the fact that many of the best vegetable sources of protein are also on the list of high-goitrogenic foods.

Still, there are a few high-protein vegetables allowed on the diet, such as mushrooms, artichokes, parsley, zucchini, beet greens, squash, and asparagus. Unfortunately, these vegetables may not contain enough protein to meet your daily recommended value. An alternative is to add a vegetarian or vegan protein powder to your daily diet. You can blend the protein powder with fresh fruits and vegetables to make a tasty smoothie for a snack or a meal replacement. You will find recipes for a number of vegan and vegetarian protein shakes and smoothies in the chapter on snacks beginning on page 175. Aside from making sure that your daily protein needs are being met, following the Hashimoto's diet as a vegan or vegetarian is actually fairly simple. Many of the recipes in this book can be modified to be vegan or vegetarian. For example, riced cauliflower (enjoyed in moderation) or diced zucchini makes a great substitute for ground meat, and portobello mushrooms can be cut into thick slices and used as a replacement for sliced meats. Chopped pumpkin or butternut squash can be used as a replacement for chopped meats in soups, stews, and other dishes. It may take a bit of creativity on your part, but there is no reason you can't succeed with the Hashimoto's diet as a vegan or vegetarian.

SOME SPECIAL INGREDIENTS

Now that you understand the Hashimoto's diet plan, you are almost ready to get into the recipes! Before you do, however, take a moment to familiarize yourself with some of the ingredients you will be using. Because the Hashimoto's diet does not allow for certain baking and cooking staples like eggs (for at least 30 days), traditional flour, and sugar, you will find a number of substitutions in the recipes. Here is an overview of some of the ingredients you may not be familiar with.

AGAR-AGAR — Also known simply as agar, this is a jelly-like substance made from seaweed and is commonly used as a vegetarian and vegan substitute for gelatin. It serves as the sole egg replacer in these recipes. Common egg replacers are made from flaxseed, which is not allowed on the Hashimoto's diet. The recipes call for agar-agar flakes, which can be blended with water into a gel-like egg replacer. If you can only find agar powder, use it at a ratio of 1 teaspoon to 1 tablespoon called for in the recipe.

COCONUT FLOUR — Because the Hashimoto's diet does not allow grains, nuts, or seeds, the best flour substitute is coconut flour. Usually white to light brown, coconut flour has a distinct coconut smell, although the flavor is typically very subtle. Coconut flour is highly absorbent, so more liquid and egg replacer are needed to bind the ingredients together than is the case with traditional flour.

COCONUT MILK — Be sure to use canned coconut milk and to shake the can before opening to mix together the solids and the liquid. Canned coconut milk is generally unsweetened and available in full-fat or lite versions. It is preferable to the coconut milk beverage that comes in a carton for cooking because it is thicker and higher in healthy fats.

COCONUT OIL—Coconut oil is solid at room temperature, which is why many of the recipes call for it to be melted. Look for cold-processed, organic coconut oil, if you can find it.

IODIZED SALT—It is best to use iodized salt rather than sea salt because iodine is an important mineral for managing the thyroid. The exception to this rule is using sea salt in fermentation and pickling recipes because sea salt is required.

PROTEIN POWDER—When choosing a protein powder for use with the Hashimoto's diet you have several options to consider. Various Paleo protein powders made with whey protein hydrolysate or whey protein isolate may be a good choice because they are the purest forms of protein and contain a high percentage of protein by weight. Even though these protein powders are made from milk proteins, the lactose and casein have been removed so they are unlikely to trigger food sensitivities or allergies. Collagen protein powder is also a good option because it is easy to digest and it provides additional support for the digestive systems and the immune system. For vegans and vegetarians, pea protein is the best option because it is made from green peas. With any commercial protein powder you may need to make some compromises and you will need to test the powders yourself to make sure you do not have a negative reaction to them.

PURE MAPLE SYRUP—Maple syrup is probably nothing new to you, but it is important that you use pure maple syrup. The pure product is all-natural, whereas bottles labeled "pancake syrup" or "breakfast syrup" usually contain high-fructose corn syrup and other artificial additives.

RAW HONEY—Raw honey is the pure, unpasteurized, unprocessed honey that comes from a honeycomb. This type of honey is available in either solid or liquid form and typically has a milky, almost yellow color rather than the rich brown color of processed honey. If you buy raw honey in solid form, you may need to melt it for certain recipes.

You are finally ready to move on to the recipes! All of the recipes in this book are designed to adhere to the dietary guidelines and food lists in this chapter. They are Paleo and gluten-free, plus many of them come with options to make them vegan- or vegetarian-friendly.

PART III
HASHIMOTO'S DIET RECIPES

CHAPTER 6
Breakfast

PALEO PUMPKIN PORRIDGE

The Hashimoto's diet excludes everything you might normally use to make granola, porridge, and other breakfast cereals. If you are a fan of hot breakfast cereals, give this Paleo pumpkin porridge a try.

Makes 4 to 6 (1-cup) servings

1 tablespoon grass-fed ghee

1 (15-ounce) can pumpkin puree

¾ cup canned coconut milk

1 tablespoon pumpkin pie spice

2 tablespoons agar-agar flakes

2 tablespoons warm water

½ cup sifted coconut flour

1 tablespoon raw honey (optional)

1. Melt the ghee in a medium saucepan over medium heat. Whisk in the pumpkin puree, coconut milk, and pumpkin pie spice, and let simmer for 5 minutes.

2. Meanwhile, whisk together the agar-agar flakes and water in a medium bowl. Whisk the agar-agar mixture and the coconut flour into the pumpkin mixture in the saucepan.

3. Simmer until thick and hot, about 3 to 4 minutes, then stir in the honey, if using. Let cook for 1 to 2 minutes more, then spoon into individual bowls and serve hot.

HOMEMADE COCONUT YOGURT

Not only is coconut yogurt dairy-free and Paleo, but it offers many benefits over traditional yogurt. Rich in protein and dietary fiber, coconut yogurt is a natural probiotic food that helps to support a healthy digestive system. Making your own coconut yogurt ensures that it will not contain any artificial ingredients and you can taste the yogurt as it ferments until it reaches the desired flavor. Enjoy it topped with fresh fruit.

Makes 8 (½-cup) servings

2 (14-ounce) cans coconut milk

½ tablespoon agar-agar flakes

¼ cup store-bought organic unsweetened coconut milk yogurt

1–2 tablespoons pure maple syrup (optional)

1. Fill a large stockpot a little more than halfway with water. Bring the water to a boil over high heat, then reduce to a simmer.

2. Place two open pint jars and their tops in the simmering water, and make sure they are immersed. Simmer for 5 to 10 minutes to sterilize the jars, then remove from the pot and let air-dry.

3. Pour the coconut milk into a medium saucepan over medium heat, and whisk until smooth. Whisk in the agar-agar flakes, then reduce the heat to low. Simmer for 5 to 10 minutes, stirring occasionally, until thick. Remove from the heat, and cool at room temperature until it reaches 100°F (measure with a candy thermometer).

4. Whisk in the store-bought coconut yogurt to add probiotic cultures. Add the maple syrup, if using, and stir well.

5. Pour the mixture into the two sterilized jars, and secure the lids tightly.

6. Fill the sink with water and add hot water to bring it to a temperature of 100°F. Place in the hot water bath, and maintain at 100°F for 12 to 24 hours by adding more hot water as needed to maintain the temperature. Taste the yogurt after 12 hours for

flavor and texture—the yogurt will thicken the longer you let it set.

7. Transfer to the refrigerator, and chill until thickened, at least 6 hours.

SAUSAGE AND SWEET POTATO HASH

Sweet potatoes are an excellent source of dietary fiber as well as vitamin C, manganese, and vitamin B6. In this recipe, you will find that tender sweet potatoes make for a tasty hash when combined with carrots, onion, and fresh garlic.

Makes 4 to 6 (1-cup) servings

2 tablespoons coconut oil

1 large yellow onion, sliced

2 cloves garlic, minced

½ pound grass-fed ground pork sausage, crumbled

1 pound sweet potatoes, peeled and chopped

2 large carrots, peeled and chopped

1 tablespoon extra virgin olive oil

2 tablespoons chopped fresh rosemary

2 teaspoons chopped fresh thyme

iodized salt and pepper

1. Melt the coconut oil in a heavy skillet over medium heat. Add the onion and garlic, then season with salt and pepper to taste. Reduce the heat to low, and cook for 20 to 30 minutes, until the onion is caramelized. Set aside in a small bowl.

2. Preheat the oven to 425°F, and line a rimmed baking sheet with foil.

3. Reheat the skillet over medium heat. Cook the sausage until evenly browned, about 5 minutes, then use a slotted spoon to transfer to a large bowl.

4. Add the caramelized onion to the bowl with the sausage, and add the sweet potatoes and carrots. Drizzle with the olive oil, and toss with the rosemary and thyme. Spread the mixture on the baking sheet.

5. Roast for 30 to 35 minutes, until the sweet potatoes and carrots are tender. Serve hot.

GOITROGEN ALERT:
max 6 to 8 servings
per week

GINGER APPLE PORK BREAKFAST SAUSAGE

Filled with morsels of tender apple, flavored with fresh garlic, and loaded with protein, this breakfast sausage is a power-packed morning meal.

Makes 6 to 8 (2-patty) servings

1 tablespoon coconut oil

1 medium sweet onion, diced

1 medium sweet apple, shredded or diced

1 tablespoon grated fresh ginger

1 clove garlic, minced

2 pounds grass-fed ground pork

2 teaspoons apple cider vinegar

1–2 teaspoons raw honey (optional)

iodized salt and pepper

1. Preheat the oven to 350°F, and line a baking sheet with foil.

2. Heat the coconut oil in a medium skillet over medium-high heat. Add the onion, apple, ginger, and garlic. Season with salt and pepper to taste. Cook until the onion is translucent, about 4 to 5 minutes.

3. Transfer the mixture to a food processor, and blend until smooth. Add the ground pork, cider vinegar, and honey, if using. Pulse until the mixture comes together.

4. Shape by hand into round 2-inch balls, then flatten into patties. Arrange on the baking sheet. Bake for 25 to 30 minutes, until cooked through.

BACON-LOADED BREAKFAST SAUSAGE

If you're looking for a hot and hearty breakfast option that isn't as carb-heavy as pancakes or muffins, try this breakfast sausage. Featuring grass-fed ground pork and uncured bacon, the dish is a protein-packed breakfast dream.

Makes 6 to 8 (2-patty) servings

6 slices grass-fed, uncured bacon

1 large yellow onion, diced

2 cloves garlic, minced

1 tablespoon pure maple syrup

1 teaspoon iodized salt

¼ teaspoon fresh ground pepper

2 pounds grass-fed ground pork

1. Preheat the oven to 350°F, and line a baking sheet with foil.

2. In a large skillet over medium-high, cook the bacon until crisp, about 3 to 4 minutes. Transfer to paper towels to drain, then chop well.

3. Combine the onion, garlic, maple syrup, salt, and pepper in a food processor. Blend until thoroughly combined, then add the ground pork and chopped bacon. Pulse several times until the mixture comes together.

4. Shape by hand into 2-inch small balls, and flatten into patties. Arrange on the baking sheet.

5. Bake for 25 to 30 minutes, until the edges are brown and the sausage is cooked through.

BLUEBERRY MAPLE BACON MEATBALLS

Blueberries and bacon may not seem like an appetizing combination, but the sweetness of the blueberries perfectly complements the savory, salty bacon. Enjoy these meatballs with a fresh breakfast smoothie to get your day started with both protein and fiber.

Makes 15 to 18 (2-meatball) servings

4 slices grass-fed, uncured bacon

1 cup fresh blueberries, rinsed well

1 small shallot, diced

1 inch fresh ginger, peeled and grated

1–2 tablespoons chopped fresh cilantro

½ pound grass-fed ground pork

½ pound grass-fed lean ground beef

1 tablespoon pure maple syrup

½ teaspoon iodized salt

¼ teaspoon pepper

1. Preheat the oven to 375°F. Line a baking sheet with foil, and spray with olive oil cooking spray.

2. In a large skillet over medium heat, cook the bacon until crisp, about 3 to 4 minutes. Transfer to paper towels to drain, then crumble into pieces.

3. Place the blueberries in a food processor, and pulse several times until chopped. Add the shallot, ginger, and cilantro, and pulse to combine. Transfer the mixture to a large bowl, and mix in the ground pork, ground beef, maple syrup, salt, and pepper by hand. Roll by hand into 1-inch meatballs, and place on the baking sheet.

4. Bake for about 8 minutes, then rotate the pan and bake for another 6 to 10 minutes, until cooked through.

COCONUT FLOUR BISCUITS

Made with just a few simple ingredients, these biscuits are sure to become a breakfast favorite, especially when you serve them with homemade Sausage and Mushroom Gravy (page 73). If you like your biscuits crunchy, bake them until they are thoroughly browned around the edges. For softer biscuits, lower the oven temperature by a few degrees or cut the cooking time short by a minute or so.

Makes 8 to 10 (1-biscuit) servings

¼ cup agar-agar flakes

¼ cup warm water

¼ cup plus 2 tablespoons sifted coconut flour

¼ cup plus 1 tablespoons melted coconut oil

2 tablespoons pure maple syrup

¾ teaspoon baking powder

pinch of iodized salt

1. Preheat the oven to 400°F, and line a baking sheet with parchment paper.

2. Whisk together the agar-agar flakes and warm water in a medium bowl, and set aside. Combine the coconut flour, coconut oil, maple syrup, baking powder, and salt in a food processor. Pulse several times to combine. Add the agar-agar mixture, and blend until smooth.

3. Once a smooth dough forms, shape by hand into 8 to 10 even-sized balls. Place on the baking sheet, and gently press by hand to about ½ inch thick.

4. Bake for 12 to 15 minutes, until the edges of the biscuits are browned. Serve warm.

SAUSAGE AND MUSHROOM GRAVY

This thick, hearty gravy pairs nicely with a batch of homemade Coconut Flour Biscuits (page 72). The gravy is guaranteed to keep you feeling full all morning long, in addition to offering good nutritional value. The mushrooms in the gravy are a rich source of iron and calcium—they are also one of the few food sources of vitamin D—and the sausage contributes protein.

Makes 6 to 8 (½-cup) servings

1 pound grass-fed ground, loose pork sausage

2 cups diced cremini mushrooms

1 teaspoon chopped fresh thyme

1 teaspoon chopped fresh rosemary

½ teaspoon dried sage

1 (14-ounce) can coconut milk

3–5 teaspoons arrowroot powder

iodized salt and pepper

1. Cook the sausage in a large skillet over medium-high heat. Stir occasionally, until fully browned, about 5 minutes, then drain the excess fat. Stir in the mushrooms, and cook until tender, about 3 to 4 minutes. Add the thyme, rosemary, and sage, then season with salt and pepper to taste.

2. Stir in the coconut milk, then add the arrowroot powder a little at a time until the gravy reaches the right thickness. Simmer over low heat for 5 to 10 minutes, until hot and thick.

3. Adjust the seasoning to taste, and serve hot with fresh biscuits.

SPICED ZUCCHINI MUFFINS

Studded with tender zucchini and spiced with ground cinnamon, these muffins are a satisfying way to start your day. Pair the muffins with homemade Ginger Apple Pork Breakfast Sausage (page 69) or Bacon-Loaded Breakfast Sausage (page 70) for a nutritionally balanced morning meal.

Makes 12 (1-muffin) servings

1½ cups shredded or grated zucchini

¼ cup plus 2 tablespoons agar-agar flakes

¼ cup plus 2 tablespoons warm water

¾ cup sifted coconut flour

1 teaspoon baking soda

1½ teaspoons ground cinnamon

¼ teaspoon iodized salt

½ cup raw honey

¼ cup melted coconut oil

1½ teaspoons vanilla extract

1. Preheat the oven to 350°F, and line a regular 12-cup muffin pan with paper liners.

2. Spread the zucchini on a clean dish towel, roll it up, and wring out as much moisture as you can.

3. Whisk together the agar-agar flakes and water in a large bowl, then set aside. Combine the coconut flour, baking soda, cinnamon, and salt in a separate medium bowl. Whisk the honey, coconut oil, and vanilla extract into the agar-agar mixture.

4. Add the dry ingredients to the wet, stirring until smooth. Fold in the shredded zucchini.

5. Spoon the batter into the muffin pan, filling each cup about three-quarters full.

6. Bake for 22 to 28 minutes until a knife inserted in the center comes out clean. Remove from the oven, and cool in the pan for about 15 minutes. Then turn out onto a wire rack to cool completely.

CINNAMON APPLESAUCE MUFFINS

Made with unsweetened applesauce in place of oil, these muffins are surprisingly healthy. Serve them up warm with a little bit of grass-fed ghee, or drizzle them with pure maple syrup for some added sweetness.

Makes 12 (1-muffin) servings

¼ cup agar-agar flakes

¼ cup warm water

½ cup sifted coconut flour

½ tablespoon ground cinnamon

1¼ teaspoons baking soda

¾ teaspoon baking powder

¼ teaspoon iodized salt

1 cup unsweetened applesauce

¼ cup melted coconut oil

1–2 tablespoons pure maple syrup

1½ teaspoons vanilla extract

1. Preheat the oven to 350°F, and line a regular 12-cup muffin pan with paper liners.

2. Whisk together the agar-agar flakes and warm water in a medium bowl, then set aside. In a separate medium bowl, combine the coconut flour, cinnamon, baking soda, baking powder, and salt. In a large bowl, whisk together the applesauce, coconut oil, maple syrup, and vanilla extract.

3. Whisk the agar-agar mixture and the dry ingredients into the applesauce mixture until smooth and lump-free.

4. Spoon the batter into the muffin pan, filling each cup about three-quarters full.

5. Bake for 22 to 28 minutes, until a knife inserted in the center comes out clean. Remove from the oven, and cool in the pan for 15 minutes. Then turn out onto a wire rack to cool completely.

CARROT GINGER MUFFINS

There is just something about the combination of carrot and ginger—the two ingredients were meant to be together! Full of fresh ginger flavor and loaded with tender shredded carrot, these vegan muffins offer a big dose of dietary fiber to start your day.

Makes 12 (1-muffin) servings

1 cup finely shredded carrot

¼ cup plus 2 tablespoons agar-agar flakes

¼ cup plus 2 tablespoons warm water

½ cup sifted coconut flour

½ teaspoon baking powder

½ teaspoon ground cinnamon

¼ teaspoon ground ginger

¼ teaspoon iodized salt

¼ cup pure maple syrup

¼ cup melted coconut oil

1 teaspoon vanilla extract

1. Preheat the oven to 350°F, and line a regular 12-cup muffin pan with paper liners.

2. Spread the shredded carrot on a clean towel, roll it up, and wring out as much moisture as you can.

3. Whisk together the agar-agar flakes and water in a large bowl and set aside.

4. In a medium bowl, whisk together the coconut flour, baking powder, cinnamon, ginger, and salt.

5. Add the maple syrup, coconut oil, and vanilla extract to the agar-agar mixture, and whisk until well combined. Stir the dry ingredients into the wet until smooth, then fold in the shredded carrot.

6. Spoon the batter into the muffin pan, filling each cup about three-quarters full.

7. Bake for 22 to 28 minutes, until a knife inserted in the center comes out clean. Remove from the oven, and cool in the pan for 15 minutes. Then turn out onto a wire rack to cool completely.

MAPLE CINNAMON WAFFLES

You may be surprised to learn that you can enjoy waffles while following the Hashimoto's diet. By swapping coconut flour for traditional all-purpose flour and using maple syrup as a natural sweetener, this recipe is Paleo, gluten-free, grain-free, and vegan.

Makes 4 (1-waffle) servings

¼ cup plus 2 tablespoons agar-agar flakes

¼ cup plus 2 tablespoons warm water

½ cup sifted coconut flour

½ teaspoon baking powder

1 teaspoon ground cinnamon

½ teaspoon iodized salt

½ cup canned coconut milk

¼ cup melted coconut oil

2 tablespoons pure maple syrup

1 tablespoon vanilla extract

1. Whisk together the agar-agar flakes and water in a medium bowl. Set aside.

2. Preheat your waffle iron according to the manufacturer's directions, and spray with olive oil cooking spray.

3. Combine the coconut flour, baking powder, cinnamon, and salt in a medium bowl. In a large bowl, beat together the coconut milk, coconut oil, maple syrup, and vanilla extract.

4. Whisk the agar-agar mixture and the dry ingredients into the coconut milk mixture until smooth. Let the batter sit at room temperature for 5 to 10 minutes to thicken.

5. Spoon the batter into the preheated waffle iron, using about ¼ to ⅓ cup according to the manufacturer's directions. Close the waffle iron, and cook until the waffle is crisp and browned.

6. Transfer to a plate and place in the oven on low heat to keep warm, and repeat with the remaining batter.

SIMPLE COCONUT FLOUR PANCAKES

Sometimes the simple things in life give us the greatest pleasure, and these simple coconut flour pancakes are no exception. Feel free blend some fresh or dried fruit into the batter or drizzle your pancakes with a natural sweetener like raw honey or pure maple syrup.

Makes 4 (2- or 3-pancake) servings

¼ cup agar-agar flakes

¼ cup warm water

1 (14-ounce) can coconut milk

¾ cup sifted coconut flour

1 tablespoon vanilla extract

1½ teaspoons baking powder

½ teaspoon iodized salt

1. Combine the agar-agar flakes and water in a medium bowl, whisking until well combined.

2. Place the coconut milk, coconut flour, vanilla extract, baking soda, and salt in a food processor. Blend for 20 seconds. Add the agar-agar mixture, and blend until smooth.

3. Preheat a large nonstick skillet or griddle pan over medium-high heat.

4. Spoon the batter into the preheated pan, using 2 to 3 tablespoons per pancake. Let cook for 2 to 3 minutes, until the underside is browned. Carefully flip the pancakes, and cook for another 1 to 2 minutes, until browned underneath.

5. Transfer to a plate and place in the oven on low heat to keep warm, repeat with the remaining batter.

6. Drizzle with maple syrup or raw honey, and serve hot.

SPICED BANANA RAISIN BREAD

Don't throw those blackened bananas away! Overripe bananas are perfect for recipes like this one because they give the bread a naturally sweet flavor while keeping it moist.

Makes 10 to 12 (1-slice) servings

1 cup sifted coconut flour

½ tablespoon ground cinnamon

1 teaspoon baking soda

½ teaspoon iodized salt

¼ cup agar-agar flakes

¼ cup warm water

¼ cup pure maple syrup

¼ cup melted coconut oil, plus more for greasing the pan

1 tablespoon vanilla extract

3 large overripe bananas, mashed

¾ cup seedless raisins

1. Preheat the oven to 325°F. Line the bottom of a standard loaf pan with parchment paper, and grease the sides with coconut oil.

2. Combine the coconut flour, cinnamon, baking soda, and salt in a medium bowl. In a large bowl, whisk together the agar-agar flakes and the warm water. Whisk the maple syrup, coconut oil, and vanilla extract into the agar-agar mixture, then stir in the mashed bananas.

3. Stir the dry ingredients into the wet until a smooth batter forms, then fold in the raisins.

4. Spread the batter in the prepared pan as evenly as possible. Bake for 55 to 60 minutes, until a knife inserted in the center comes out clean.

5. Cool the bread for 15 minutes in the pan, then turn out onto a wire rack to cool completely.

BLUEBERRY CINNAMON PANCAKES

The perfect combination of tender pancakes and sweet blueberries, this is one breakfast you definitely don't want to miss. If you have never tried the flavor combination of blueberry and cinnamon, you are in for a treat! Serve these pancakes drizzled with pure maple syrup.

Makes 4 (2- to 3-pancake) servings

¼ cup agar-agar flakes

¼ cup plus 2 tablespoons warm water

1½ cups canned coconut milk

1 tablespoon vanilla extract

1 cup sifted coconut flour

2 teaspoons baking powder

1 teaspoon ground cinnamon

½ teaspoon iodized salt

1–2 cups fresh blueberries

1. Whisk together the agar-agar flakes and warm water in a large bowl. Add the coconut milk and vanilla extract, and whisk until smooth. Whisk in the coconut flour, baking powder, cinnamon, and salt until no lumps remain.

2. Preheat a large nonstick skillet or griddle pan over medium-high heat.

3. Spoon the batter into the pan, using 2 to 3 tablespoons per pancake. Sprinkle a few fresh blueberries into the wet batter, and cook until the underside is browned, about 1 to 2 minutes.

4. Carefully flip the pancakes, and cook for another minute or so, until browned underneath.

5. Transfer to a plate and place in the oven on low heat to keep warm, and repeat with the remaining batter.

COCONUT FLOUR PUMPKIN BREAD

This pumpkin bread is lightly sweetened and simply divine when served with a little ghee. Along with being delicious, it is packed with healthy gluten-free and grain-free carbohydrates.

Makes 8 to 10 (1-slice) servings

¼ cup plus 1 tablespoon agar-agar flakes

¼ cup plus 1 tablespoon warm water

1 cup pumpkin puree

¼ cup pure maple syrup

¼ cup melted coconut oil, plus more to grease the pan

1 teaspoon vanilla extract

½ cup sifted coconut flour

1½ tablespoons pumpkin pie spice

1 teaspoon baking powder

½ teaspoon iodized salt

1. Preheat the oven to 400°F, and grease a regular loaf pan with coconut oil.

2. Whisk together the agar-agar flakes and warm water in a medium bowl. In a large bowl, whisk together the pumpkin puree, maple syrup, coconut oil, and vanilla extract. In a small bowl, whisk together the coconut flour, pumpkin pie spice, baking soda, and salt.

3. Whisk the dry ingredients and the agar-agar mixture into the pumpkin mixture. Stir until smooth.

4. Spread the batter into the loaf pan as evenly as possible. Bake for 20 to 25 minutes, until a knife inserted in the center comes out clean.

5. Cool the bread for 15 minutes in the pan, then turn out onto a wire rack to cool completely.

CHAPTER 7
Lunch

COCONUT-CRUSTED CHICKEN STRIPS WITH GARLIC DIPPING SAUCE

Serve these tender, crispy, coconut-coated chicken strips with home-made garlic dipping sauce or enjoy them atop a fresh green salad.
Makes 4 to 6 (4-strip) servings

4 free-range boneless, skinless chicken breasts

3 tablespoons agar-agar flakes

3 tablespoons warm water

¼ cup canned coconut milk

¾ cup sifted coconut flour

2 cups unsweetened shredded coconut

1. Preheat the oven to 400°F, and line a rimmed baking sheet with parchment paper.

2. Lay the chicken breasts flat on a sheet of waxed paper, and cover with another sheet. Use a meat mallet to flatten the chicken breasts to about ½ inch thick. Cut into strips about 1 inch wide, and set aside.

3. Whisk together the agar-agar flakes and water in a medium bowl, then whisk in the coconut milk.

4. Place the coconut flour in a shallow dish, and the shredded coconut in a separate shallow dish.

5. Dredge the chicken strips one at a time in the coconut flour, then dip in the coconut milk mixture. Place in the shredded coconut, and press down to coat both sides.

6. Arrange on the baking sheet. Bake for 10 to 12 minutes, until the chicken is cooked through and the coconut is browned.

GARLIC DIPPING SAUCE
Makes 1 cup

1 cup canned coconut milk

¼ cup extra virgin olive oil

4 cloves garlic, minced

¼ teaspoon salt

1. Combine all of the ingredients in a blender.

2. Blend on high speed for 2 to 3 minutes until thick and blended. Spoon into a bowl and serve with coconut-crusted chicken strips for dipping.

CURRY ROASTED BUTTERNUT SQUASH SOUP

This butternut squash soup is seasoned with curry powder to give it a unique, earthy flavor and it is blended with coconut milk for a creamy finish. In addition to being an excellent source of gluten-free and grain-free carbs, butternut squash is naturally rich in potassium. It is also rich in vitamin B6, which plays an important role in both immune function and nervous system health.

Makes 4 to 6 (1-cup) servings

2 (2-pound) butternut squash

olive oil, as needed

1 tablespoon coconut oil

1 medium yellow onion, sliced

2 cloves garlic, minced

1 tablespoon curry powder

3 cups chicken broth

1 (14-ounce) can coconut milk

iodized salt and pepper

1. Preheat the oven to 350°F, and line a baking sheet with foil.

2. Cut each squash in half, then scoop out and discard the seeds. Place cut side down on the baking sheet, and drizzle with olive oil. Roast for 35 to 40 minutes, until tender. Remove and set aside.

3. Heat the coconut oil in a large saucepan over medium-high heat. Add the onion, and cook until translucent, about 4 to 5 minutes. Stir in the garlic and curry powder, then cook for another minute or so until fragrant.

4. When the squash is cool enough, remove the peel and chop the flesh. Add the squash and the chicken broth to the saucepan. Season with salt and pepper to taste. Bring to a simmer, and cook on low for 20 minutes.

5. Remove from the heat, and puree with an immersion blender until smooth. Whisk in the coconut milk, and adjust the seasoning to taste. Serve hot.

CHILLED AVOCADO LIME SOUP

This is a really refreshing soup for a hot summer day. Garnish it with chopped fresh cilantro and crumbled bacon or, for a vegan- and vegetarian-friendly version, top with grated fresh coconut or diced fresh mango in place of the bacon.

Makes 4 (1-cup) servings

2 large ripe avocados, chopped

1 cup chopped fresh cilantro, plus extra for garnish

2 cloves garlic, minced

1½ cups vegetable broth

1 cup canned coconut milk

¼ cup fresh lime juice (from about 2 large limes)

iodized salt and pepper

crumbled bacon

1. Place the avocado, cilantro, and garlic in a blender. Pulse several times to chop. Add the vegetable broth, coconut milk, and lime juice, then blend at high speed until smooth and well combined.

2. Add water, if needed, to thin the soup to the desired consistency. Season with salt and pepper to taste.

3. Pour into a large bowl, cover with plastic wrap, and chill in the refrigerator for several hours before serving.

CREAMY SAFFRON CARROT SOUP

This saffron carrot soup combines the subtle honey-like flavor of saffron with the earthy sweetness of carrots and leeks, all blended into a creamy concoction. Carrots are rich in beta-carotene, a powerful antioxidant that helps to protect cells against free-radical damage, and saffron is an herbal flower with a delicate flavor and its own antioxidant benefits.

Makes 4 to 6 (1-cup) servings

2 tablespoons coconut oil

2 medium leeks, chopped (white and light green parts only)

3 cloves garlic, minced

1 pound carrots, peeled and sliced

1 pound sweet potatoes, peeled and chopped

pinch of saffron

5 cups vegetable broth

½ cup canned coconut milk

iodized salt and pepper

1. Melt the coconut oil in a large saucepan over medium heat. Add the leeks and garlic, and cook for 6 to 8 minutes, stirring often, until the leeks are softened. Stir in the carrots and sweet potatoes, then sauté for 2 to 3 minutes before adding the saffron and the vegetable broth. Bring the mixture to a boil, then reduce the heat and simmer for 15 to 20 minutes, until the vegetables are tender.

2. Remove from the heat. Puree with an immersion blender until smooth. Whisk in the coconut milk, and season with salt and pepper to taste. Add more broth, if needed, to thin the soup to the desired consistency. Serve hot.

GOITROGEN ALERT:
max 6 to 8 servings
per week

THAI COCONUT CHICKEN SOUP

This Thai-inspired chicken soup has just the right amount of coconut flavor, which blends perfectly with fresh lime zest and tender shiitake mushrooms.

Makes 4 to 6 (1-cup) servings

1 tablespoon coconut oil

1 small yellow onion, chopped

2 tablespoons grated fresh ginger

1 tablespoon minced fresh garlic

1 large carrot, peeled and grated

1 cup sliced shiitake mushrooms

1 bunch fresh green onions, white and green parts, cut into 1-inch pieces

1¼ pounds free-range, boneless, skinless chicken breast, chopped

4 cups chicken broth

1 (14-ounce) can coconut milk

3 teaspoons fish sauce

¼ cup chopped fresh cilantro

1 teaspoon fresh lime zest

iodized salt and pepper

basil, sliced

1. Heat the coconut oil in a large saucepan over medium heat. Add the onion, ginger, and garlic, and cook for 4 to 5 minutes, until the onions are translucent. Stir in the carrot, mushrooms, and green onions, and cook for 4 minutes.

2. Push the vegetables to the side of the saucepan, then add the chopped chicken. Cook for 1 minute without stirring. Then stir in the chicken broth, coconut milk, and fish sauce. Bring to a simmer, reduce the heat, and cook on low for 15 to 20 minutes, until the chicken is cooked through.

3. Stir in the cilantro and lime zest, then season with salt and pepper to taste.

4. Spoon the soup into individual bowls, and garnish with sliced basil.

CREAM OF CHICKEN SOUP WITH VEGGIES

Simple to prepare, this dish is full of tender veggies and hearty chicken. If you prefer a creamier soup, puree the mixture in the blender before you add the chicken.

Makes 6 (1-cup) servings

2 tablespoons coconut oil

1 medium yellow onion, chopped

2 medium carrots, peeled and chopped

2 stalks celery, thickly sliced

½ cup arrowroot powder

½ cup cool water

6 cups chicken broth

1 medium bay leaf

¼ cup chopped fresh parsley

1 teaspoon chopped fresh thyme

1 (14-ounce) can coconut milk

2 free-range, boneless, skinless chicken breasts, cooked and shredded

iodized salt and pepper

1. Melt the coconut oil in a large saucepan over medium heat. Add the onion, carrots, and celery, and cook for 12 to 15 minutes, until softened.

2. Whisk together the arrowroot powder and water in a small bowl.

3. Stir the chicken broth and the arrowroot powder mixture into the saucepan. Add the bay leaf, parsley, and thyme, then season with salt and pepper to taste.

4. Bring the mixture to a simmer, then reduce the heat and simmer for 15 minutes. Stir in the coconut milk and the shredded chicken. Cook for another 5 minutes, or until the chicken is heated through.

5. Adjust the seasoning to taste, and discard the bay leaf. Serve hot.

SLOW COOKER HEARTY CHICKEN BACON CHOWDER

This hearty chowder is thick, rich, and loaded with bacon flavor. All you have to do is throw the ingredients together in your slow cooker with minimal preparation, and the slow cooker will do the rest. Serve the chowder hot, garnished with crumbled bacon and sliced green onions.

Makes 6 to 8 (1-cup) servings

8 ounces cremini mushrooms, thinly sliced

1 medium yellow onion, chopped

2 stalks celery, chopped

1 medium leek, chopped (white and light green parts only)

1 tablespoon minced fresh garlic

4 tablespoons coconut oil, divided

2 cups chicken broth, divided

2 free-range, boneless, skinless chicken breasts

2 (14-ounce) cans coconut milk

2 teaspoons chopped fresh thyme

1 pound uncured bacon, chopped, plus more for garnish

iodized salt and pepper

2 sliced green onions, white and green parts, for garnish

1. Combine the mushrooms, onion, celery, leek, and garlic in the bottom of a slow cooker. Top the vegetables with 2 tablespoons of coconut oil, then season with salt and pepper to taste. Pour in 1 cup of chicken broth, cover, and cook on low for 1 hour.

2. During the last 15 minutes of cook time, heat the remaining 2 tablespoons of coconut oil in a large skillet over medium-high heat. Season the chicken breasts with salt and pepper, and add them to the skillet. Cook for 4 to 5 minutes on each side, until browned, then remove to a cutting board.

3. Pour the remaining 1 cup of chicken broth into the skillet, and scrape any browned bits from the bottom of the pan. Simmer for 1 to 2 minutes, then pour the skillet contents into the slow cooker. Add the coconut milk and thyme to the slow cooker, and stir until well combined.

4. Cut the chicken into bite-size chunks. Add the chicken and the uncooked chopped bacon to the slow cooker. Stir to thoroughly combine, cover, and cook on low for 6 to 8 hours, until thick and heated through.

5. Cook the remaining bacon in a small skillet over medium-high heat until crisp, about 4 to 5 minutes, then drain on paper towels. Serve the soup hot, garnished with sliced green onion and crumbled bacon.

CREAMY MUSHROOM BISQUE

Tender mushrooms in a thick, creamy broth makes for a delicious lunch. Not only are mushrooms an excellent source of vitamin D, but they are rich in antioxidants, amino acids, and natural antibiotic compounds.

Makes 4 to 6 (1-cup) servings

3 tablespoons coconut oil

1 large yellow onion, diced

2 pounds mixed mushrooms, sliced

1½ teaspoons chopped fresh rosemary

1 teaspoon chopped fresh thyme

8 cups vegetable broth

1 (14-ounce) can coconut milk

½ cup chopped fresh parsley

iodized salt and pepper

1. Heat the coconut oil in a large saucepan over medium-high heat. Add the onion, and cook for 4 to 5 minutes, until translucent. Stir in the mushrooms, rosemary, and thyme, and cook for 7 to 8 minutes. Add the vegetable broth, and bring the mixture to a boil.

2. Reduce the heat, and simmer on medium-low for 12 to 15 minutes. Stir in the coconut milk, and season with salt and pepper to taste.

3. Simmer for 5 more minutes, then stir in the parsley and serve hot.

CRANBERRY ARUGULA SALAD WITH CIDER VINAIGRETTE

This salad combines the strong, slightly bitter flavor of fresh arugula and the tanginess of cranberries with a sweet apple cider vinaigrette. This salad is loaded with antioxidants and vitamins and minerals like vitamin A, vitamin C, folate, and calcium.

Makes 4 servings

¼ cup extra virgin olive oil

3 tablespoons apple cider vinegar

1½ tablespoons fresh lemon juice

1 tablespoon raw honey

1 clove garlic, minced

8 cups fresh baby arugula, rinsed and drained

1 cup thinly sliced seedless cucumber

¼ cup thinly sliced red onion

½ cup unsweetened dried cranberries

iodized salt and pepper

1. To make the vinaigrette, whisk together the olive oil, apple cider vinegar, lemon juice, honey, and garlic in a small bowl. Season with salt and pepper to taste, then let sit for 30 minutes for the flavors to combine.

2. Toss together the arugula, cucumber, and red onion in a large salad bowl. Add the vinaigrette, then toss to coat. Garnish with cranberries to serve.

GOITROGEN ALERT:
max 6 to 8 servings
per week

AVOCADO SPINACH SALAD WITH BACON DRESSING

If you think that a salad is just a pile of greens, this avocado spinach salad will change your mind. Featuring crisp baby spinach topped with tender slices of avocado and a warm bacon dressing, this is unlike any salad you've had before and you won't soon forget it.

Makes 4 servings

8 slices grass-fed, uncured bacon

¼ cup apple cider vinegar

1 tablespoon raw honey

½ teaspoon garlic powder

8 cups coarsely chopped fresh baby spinach

1 cup sliced fresh white mushrooms

½ small red onion, thinly sliced

1 large ripe avocado, thinly sliced

iodized salt and pepper

1. In a large skillet over medium-high heat, cook the bacon until crisp, about 4 to 5 minutes. Transfer to paper towels to drain, then crumble into pieces.

2. To make the dressing, spoon the grease into a measuring cup. Pour about ⅓ cup back into the skillet. Reheat the skillet over medium heat, then whisk in the apple cider vinegar, honey, and garlic powder. Season lightly with salt and pepper to taste, and cook until heated through.

3. In a large bowl, toss the spinach with the mushrooms and red onion. Divide the mixture among four salad plates. Top each salad with fresh avocado and crumbled bacon, then drizzle with the bacon dressing.

GOITROGEN ALERT:
max 6 to 8 servings
per week

GREEK-STYLE VEGETABLE SALAD

For a simple salad that's full of flavor, this vegetable salad fits the bill. Tossed in a homemade dressing flavored with plenty of fresh herbs, the salad is crisp and crunchy—everything a fresh salad should be.

Makes 4 servings

¾ cup red wine vinegar

¼ cup extra virgin olive oil

3 tablespoons fresh lemon juice

1 tablespoon fresh lemon zest

1 tablespoon chopped fresh basil

1½ teaspoons chopped fresh oregano

1½ teaspoons chopped fresh rosemary

1½ teaspoons chopped fresh thyme

4 cups chopped romaine lettuce

1 small seedless cucumber, halved lengthwise and thinly sliced

½ small red onion, thinly sliced

½ cup pitted Kalamata olives

1 (14-ounce) can artichoke hearts, drained and chopped

iodized salt and pepper

1. Whisk together the red wine vinegar, olive oil, lemon juice, and lemon zest in a large bowl. Add the basil, oregano, rosemary, and thyme, then season with salt and pepper to taste. Toss in the romaine lettuce, cucumber, red onion, olives, and artichoke hearts.

2. Divide among four salad plates, and serve immediately.

BALSAMIC GLAZED CHICKEN SPINACH SALAD

Loaded with tender spinach and mushrooms plus crunchy carrots and jicama, this fresh vegetable salad is topped with tender grilled chicken marinated in a sweet balsamic glaze. Feel free to customize this recipe with fresh spring greens and any other vegetables you have on hand, and don't be afraid to add some fresh fruit to brighten up the flavors.

Makes 4 servings

1 pound fresh spinach, stems trimmed

8 ounces white mushrooms, thinly sliced

1 carrot, peeled and grated

½ large fresh jicama, peeled and cut into matchsticks

¼ small red onion, thinly sliced

¼ cup extra virgin olive oil, plus extra to serve

¼ cup balsamic vinegar, plus extra to serve

1 teaspoon pure maple syrup

2 cloves garlic, minced

1½ pounds free-range boneless, skinless chicken breast tenders

iodized salt and pepper

1. To make the salad, combine the spinach, mushrooms, carrot, jicama, and red onion in a large bowl, and set aside.

2. To make the marinade, whisk together the olive oil, balsamic vinegar, maple syrup, and garlic in a small bowl. Season with salt and pepper to taste.

3. Place the chicken in a zip-top plastic bag, and pour in the marinade. Shake to coat the chicken, seal the bag, and refrigerate for at least 1 hour.

4. Preheat your grill to medium-high heat, and brush the grates with olive oil. If using a grill pan on the stovetop, spray with olive oil cooking spray and preheat over medium-high heat.

5. Place the chicken on the grill perpendicular to the grates. Grill for about 2 minutes, then flip the chicken, and cook for another 2 minutes, until cooked through.

6. Remove to a cutting board, and cover loosely with foil while you prepare the salad.

7. Toss the salad with the olive oil and balsamic vinegar, and divide among four salad plates. Slice the chicken, and divide evenly among the salads, laying the sliced on top. Drizzle the salads with extra virgin olive oil and balsamic vinegar, if desired, to serve.

GOITROGEN ALERT:
max 6 to 8 servings
per week

CHOPPED VEGETABLE SALAD WITH CITRUS DRESSING

A delicious blend of crisp veggies tossed in a citrus dressing, this salad is the perfect midday meal. Feel free to customize this recipe with fresh seasonal veggies from your local farmer's market.

Makes 6 (2½-cup) servings

FOR THE CITRUS DRESSING

½ cup extra virgin olive oil

2 tablespoons white wine vinegar

1½ tablespoons fresh lemon juice

1 tablespoon fresh orange juice

1 medium shallot, thinly sliced

¼ teaspoon fresh lemon zest

⅛ teaspoon ground ginger

iodized salt and pepper

FOR THE SALAD

1 large seedless cucumber, halved lengthwise and thinly sliced

2 carrots, peeled and cut into matchsticks

2 stalks celery, thinly sliced

1 small zucchini, thinly sliced

1 large fresh jicama, peeled and thinly sliced

½ small red onion, thinly sliced

6–8 cups chopped romaine lettuce

¼ cup chopped fresh basil

1. To make the dressing, whisk together the olive oil, white wine vinegar, lemon juice, and orange juice in a medium bowl. Add the shallot, lemon zest, and ginger, then season with salt and pepper to taste. Whisk until thoroughly combined. Set aside.

2. To prepare the salad, combine the cucumber, carrots, celery, zucchini, jicama, and red onion in a large bowl. Toss with dressing to taste, until evenly coated.

3. Serve the dressed vegetables over a bed of chopped lettuce, and garnish with the chopped basil.

GOITROGEN ALERT:
max 6 to 8 servings
per week

CREAMY LOBSTER AVOCADO SALAD

This indulgent salad is made with tender bites of lobster and chunks of avocado tossed in a coconut milk sauce. Serve it chilled over a bed of crisp lettuce or roll it up in a large leaf of Boston lettuce for a healthy wrap.

Makes 4 (1-cup) servings

4 (6–8-ounce) wild lobster tails, fresh or frozen and thawed

½ cup canned coconut milk

¼ cup fresh lemon juice

2 tablespoons chopped fresh chives

1 large ripe avocado, chopped

2 stalks celery, thinly sliced

iodized salt and pepper

1. Bring a large pot of salted water to a boil, and prepare an ice bath in the sink.

2. Place the lobster tails in the boiling water, and cook for 8 to 10 minutes, until the shells turn bright red. Immediately transfer to the ice water bath, and soak for 2 minutes.

3. Drain the lobster tails, then cut in half lengthwise and scoop out the meat. Chop into bite-size chunks, and pat dry with paper towels. Place in a bowl, and chill for 15 minutes while you prepare the rest of the salad.

4. Whisk together the coconut milk, lemon juice, and chives in a medium bowl. Season lightly with salt and pepper to taste. Add the avocado, celery, and chilled lobster, and toss until combined.

5. Cover the bowl with plastic wrap, and chill in the refrigerator for 15 minutes before serving.

SWEET POTATOES STUFFED WITH SLOW-COOKED PORK

Tender pulled pork atop baked sweet potatoes is the foundation for this hot and hearty meal. Top it off with homemade barbecue sauce that is made without tomatoes, making it completely nightshade-free.

Makes 4 servings

FOR THE SWEET POTATOES AND PORK

1 medium yellow onion, thinly sliced

2 cloves garlic, minced

2 pounds grass-fed boneless pork shoulder

½ cup beef broth

2 pounds sweet potatoes

sliced green onions, white and green parts only

iodized salt and pepper

FOR THE BARBECUE SAUCE

¼ cup pure maple syrup

1 tablespoon red wine vinegar

1 tablespoon fresh lemon juice

1 teaspoon garlic powder

1 teaspoon ground ginger

½ teaspoon iodized salt

1 tablespoon bacon grease or coconut oil

2 medium carrots, peeled and diced

1 medium yellow onion, diced

1 cup diced fresh strawberries

1. Spread the onion and garlic in the bottom of a slow cooker. Season the pork with salt and pepper, then place it on top of the onion and garlic. Pour in the beef broth, and cover the slow cooker. Cook on low for 7 to 8 hours, until the pork is very tender. If you don't have a slow cooker, prepare this recipe on the stovetop using a covered Dutch oven, and reduce the cook time to 2 to 3 hours.

2. Prepare the barbecue sauce by combining the maple syrup, red wine vinegar, and lemon juice in a small saucepan over medium heat. Whisk in the garlic powder, ginger, and salt. Stir in the bacon grease or coconut oil, carrots, onion, and strawberries. Simmer until the onion is very tender, about 18 to 20 minutes.

3. Spoon the mixture into a blender, and blend on high speed until smooth. Return the sauce to the saucepan, and simmer for 10 minutes. Remove from the heat, and set aside.

4. Once the pork is almost done, preheat the oven to 400°F.

5. Pierce the sweet potatoes several times with a fork, and place them in the oven on the middle rack. Bake for 45 minutes, or until tender, then remove from the oven.

6. Transfer the pork to a large bowl, and shred the meat with two forks. Add the meat back to the slow cooker and stir in the homemade barbecue sauce until thoroughly combined. Cover and cook on low for 30 minutes—if preparing in a Dutch oven on the stovetop, cook on low heat, covered, for 20 minutes.

7. Split the sweet potatoes evenly down the middle. Fill them with the pulled pork, and garnish with sliced green onions to serve.

GOITROGEN ALERT:
max 6 to 8 servings
per week

CURRIED ROOT VEGETABLE CAKES

These cakes are fried until golden brown and served with a light coconut, lemon, and dill sauce. This is a great recipe to prepare ahead of time because you can reheat the cakes in the oven until crisp.

Makes about 4 (4-cake) servings

½ cup canned coconut milk

2 tablespoons chopped fresh dill

1 tablespoon fresh lemon juice

2 cups finely shredded carrots

2 cups finely shredded beets

1 cup finely shredded parsnips

2 tablespoons agar-agar flakes

2 tablespoons warm water

½ cup sifted coconut flour

4 green onions, thinly sliced, white and green parts

1 teaspoon curry powder

2 tablespoons coconut oil, plus more as needed

iodized salt and pepper

1. To make the dill sauce, whisk together the coconut milk, dill, and lemon juice in a small bowl. Set aside.

2. Preheat the oven to 300°F, and line a baking sheet with parchment paper.

3. Spread the shredded carrots, beets, and parsnips on clean dish towels, roll them up, and wring out as much moisture as you can.

4. Whisk together the agar-agar flakes and warm water in a large bowl. Toss in the shredded vegetables, coconut flour, green onions, curry powder, and salt and pepper to taste.

5. Melt 2 tablespoons of coconut oil in a large skillet over medium-high heat. Spoon about ¼ cup of the vegetable mixture into the skillet, and spread it into a thick disc. Repeat until there is no more room in the skillet, but be sure to leave a little space between cakes. Fry for 3 to 4 minutes on each side, until crisp and browned.

6. Transfer the fried cakes to the baking sheet, and place in the oven to keep warm.

7. Repeat until all of the vegetable cakes have been fried, adding more oil to the skillet as needed. Serve warm with a dollop of the sauce.

CRISPY FRIED FISH TACOS

Fried in a crispy coconut flour batter and drizzled with coconut lime sauce, these fish tacos are served on romaine lettuce leaves instead of tortillas which use wheat or corn.

Makes 4 (1-taco) servings

½ cup canned coconut milk

¼ cup chopped fresh cilantro

2 tablespoons fresh lime juice

1 clove garlic, minced

2 tablespoons agar-agar flakes

2 tablespoons warm water

¼ cup sifted coconut flour

¼ cup sparkling water

1¼ cups arrowroot powder, divided

extra virgin olive oil, as needed

4 (6-ounce) boneless, wild tilapia fillets

2 romaine hearts, leaves separated

iodized salt and pepper

1. Make a coconut lime sauce by whisking together the coconut milk, cilantro, lime juice, and garlic in a small bowl. Set aside.

2. In a medium bowl, whisk together the agar-agar flakes and water. Stir in the coconut flour, then whisk in the sparkling water and ¾ cup of the arrowroot powder until a smooth batter forms. Season lightly with salt and pepper to taste, and set aside.

3. Fill a heavy skillet with about 1 inch of olive oil, and heat it to 350°F.

4. Rinse the fish in cool water, and pat dry with paper towels. Cut into 1-inch strips. Dredge in the remaining ½ cup of arrowroot powder, and shake off the excess. Dip the fish in the batter, letting the excess drip off. Place in the hot oil.

5. Cook for about 1 minute, then flip the fish and cook for another minute, until golden brown. Transfer to paper towels to drain, and repeat with the remaining fish and batter.

6. Serve on romaine lettuce leaves, drizzled with the sauce.

HAWAIIAN-STYLE TURKEY BURGERS

These tender grilled turkey burgers topped with fresh pineapple are finished off with a sweet mango salsa. For added depth of flavor, place the pineapple slices on the grill for a minute or two.

Makes 4 servings

1 ripe mango, diced

½ cup finely chopped seedless cucumber

¼ cup finely diced red onion

¼ cup chopped fresh cilantro

2 tablespoons chopped fresh basil

1 clove garlic, minced

¼ cup unsweetened pineapple juice

2 tablespoons coconut aminos

1 tablespoon agave

1 teaspoon garlic powder

1 teaspoon dried ginger

1½ pounds free-range, lean, ground turkey

fresh leaves of Boston lettuce

4 slices fresh pineapple

iodized salt and pepper

1. Prepare a mango salsa by tossing together the mango, cucumber, red onion, cilantro, basil, and garlic in a medium bowl. Cover with plastic wrap, and chill in the refrigerator until ready to use.

2. In a large bowl, whisk together the pineapple juice, coconut aminos, agave, garlic powder, ginger, and salt and pepper to taste. Mix in the ground turkey by hand until thoroughly combined. Divide into six even-sized patties.

3. Preheat your grill to medium heat and brush the grates with olive oil. If using a grill pan on the stovetop, spray with olive oil cooking spray and preheat over medium-high heat.

4. Place the patties on the grill, and cook for 4 to 5 minutes on each side, until the internal temperature reads 180°F. Then transfer to a cutting board, cover loosely with foil, and let rest for 5 minutes.

5. Place the burgers on several leaves of Boston lettuce layered on top of each other. Top each patty with a slice of fresh pineapple and a scoop of mango salsa.

THAI-STYLE PORK LETTUCE WRAPS

Loaded with tender ground pork flavored with fish sauce and coconut aminos, these wraps are great as a filling lunch dish but they can also be served as an appetizer. You can substitute ground turkey for a slightly leaner option, or try the recipe with ground beef. Don't skimp on the vegetable relish—its delightful crunch and tangy herb flavor is what really makes the meal!

Makes 4 (1-wrap) servings

1 head Boston lettuce

1 teaspoon coconut oil

1 medium yellow onion, diced

1 tablespoon grated fresh ginger

2 cloves garlic, minced

½ pound grass-fed ground pork

2 tablespoons coconut aminos

2 tablespoon fish sauce

1 cup finely diced seedless cucumber

1 small carrot, peeled and grated

2 tablespoons minced red onion

2 tablespoons chopped fresh cilantro

1 tablespoon chopped fresh basil

2 tablespoons fresh lime juice

1 tablespoon apple cider vinegar

1 teaspoon agave

iodized salt and pepper

1. Separate the lettuce leaves, and set aside.

2. Heat the coconut oil in a medium skillet over medium heat. Add the onion, ginger, and garlic, and cook for 4 to 5 minutes, until the onions are translucent. Stir in the ground pork, and cook until evenly browned, about 5 minutes.

3. Pour off the fat, then stir in the coconut aminos and fish sauce. Season with salt and pepper to taste. Transfer the pork mixture to a serving bowl.

4. To make the relish, toss together the cucumber, carrot, red onion, cilantro, basil, lime juice, and agave.

5. To serve, spoon the pork mixture into lettuce leaves, and top with the vegetable relish.

COCONUT FLOUR BALSAMIC VEGGIE WRAPS

With crisp veggies tossed in balsamic vinegar, these wraps are a healthy vegan and vegetarian go-to lunch. The wraps themselves are made with arrowroot powder and coconut flour, and lightly fried to make them warm and pliable.

Makes 4 servings

2½ tablespoons agar-agar flakes

½ cup warm water

2 teaspoons melted coconut oil

¼ cup plus 2 tablespoons arrowroot powder

1 tablespoon coconut flour

¼ teaspoon iodized salt

4 leaves romaine lettuce, coarsely chopped

3 tablespoons balsamic vinegar

2 tablespoons extra virgin olive oil

1 teaspoon agave

1 medium carrot, peeled and grated

1 medium stalk celery, thinly sliced

½ cup sliced mushrooms

½ cup diced jicama

¼ cup diced red onion

1. Whisk together the agar-agar flakes and warm water in a medium bowl. Add the coconut oil, and whisk until smooth. Whisk in the arrowroot powder, coconut flour, and salt until a smooth batter forms.

2. Preheat an 8-inch skillet over medium heat, and spray with olive oil cooking spray. Pour in about a quarter of the batter, and tilt the pan to spread it evenly along the bottom. Cook for 1 minute, then carefully flip the wrap and cook for 1 minute on the other side. Slide the wrap onto a plate. Repeat with the remaining batter.

3. Lay the four wraps flat, and arrange the lettuce leaves in the center of each.

4. Whisk together the balsamic vinegar, olive oil, and agave and toss with the carrot, celery, mushrooms, jicama, and red onion.

5. Lay the veggie mixture in the middle of the wraps, and roll the wraps around the filling.

CHAPTER 8
Dinner

ROSEMARY CITRUS SWORDFISH STEAKS

The flavors of fresh orange and lemon juice blend nicely with chopped rosemary in this simple dish. If you like, try this recipe with other types of lean fish, such as salmon, halibut, haddock, or pollock.

Makes 4 servings

¾ cup fresh orange juice

¼ cup fresh lemon juice

1 tablespoon fresh orange zest

2 cloves garlic, minced

2 sprigs fresh rosemary, chopped

4 (6-ounce) wild, boneless swordfish steaks

2 tablespoons coconut oil

iodized salt and pepper

1. Preheat the oven to 400°F.

2. To make the rosemary citrus sauce, whisk together the orange juice, lemon juice, orange zest, garlic, and rosemary in a small bowl. Set aside.

3. Season the swordfish steaks on both sides with salt and pepper.

4. Melt the coconut oil in a large ovenproof skillet over medium-high heat. Add the swordfish steaks, and cook for 3 minutes, until the undersides are browned.

5. Turn the steaks, and pour the sauce over them. Bring the sauce to a simmer, then transfer the skillet to the oven.

6. Bake for 5 to 8 minutes, until just cooked through. Serve hot, with a drizzle of sauce from the pan.

GRILLED SALMON FILLETS WITH BASIL ARTICHOKE PESTO

Enjoy the natural flavor of grilled salmon fillets topped with homemade pesto in this quick and easy recipe. In addition to fresh basil, the pesto includes artichokes, a natural source of dietary fiber and antioxidants. This recipe pairs well with a simple side dish like Garlic Grilled Asparagus (page 167).

Makes 4 servings (serving size is 8-ounce fillet plus 2 to 3 tablespoons pesto)

FOR THE PESTO

4 cups chopped fresh basil

¼ cup canned artichoke hearts, drained and chopped

1 tablespoon fresh lemon juice, plus more to serve

2 cloves garlic, minced

2–3 tablespoons extra virgin olive oil

iodized salt and pepper

FOR THE SALMON FILLETS

4 (8-ounce) wild, boneless salmon fillets, skin on

¼ cup fresh lemon juice

iodized salt and pepper

1. To make the pesto, place the basil and artichoke hearts in a food processor, and pulse several times to chop. Add the lemon juice, and garlic, and salt and pepper to taste, and blend to combine. With the processor running, drizzle in the olive oil until the desired consistency is reached.

2. Preheat the grill to high heat, and brush the grates with olive oil. If using a grill pan, spray with olive oil cooking spray and preheat to high heat.

3. Season the salmon with salt and pepper. Brush with lemon juice, then place on the grill, skin side up. Sear for 2 minutes with the lid closed, until grill marks appear. Flip the fillets skin side down, and grill for another 3 to 5 minutes with the lid closed, until just cooked through.

4. Transfer to a serving platter, and top with pesto to serve.

EASY BAKED COCONUT JUMBO SHRIMP

Tender shrimp in a crispy fried coconut coating is the perfect summer meal. Enjoy this dish as a hearty meal or halve the recipe to serve as an appetizer.

Makes 4 (6-ounce) servings

¼ cup plus 2 tablespoons arrowroot powder

¾ teaspoon iodized salt

¼ teaspoon fresh ground pepper

3 tablespoons agar-agar flakes

3 tablespoons warm water

1¼ cups unsweetened shredded coconut

1½ pounds wild, raw shrimp, peeled and deveined

1. Preheat the oven to 400°F, and set a wire rack over a baking sheet.

2. Combine the arrowroot powder, salt, and pepper in a medium bowl. Whisk together the agar-agar flakes and water in a separate bowl. Place the shredded coconut in a shallow dish.

3. Dredge the shrimp individually in the arrowroot mixture, then dip in the agar-agar mixture. Place in the dish with the coconut, and press to coat both sides.

4. Arrange the shrimp on the wire rack, and place the baking sheet in the oven. Bake until golden brown, about 10 minutes on each side, and serve hot out of the oven.

STEAMED MUSSELS IN LEMON GARLIC BROTH

Mussels are an extra-lean source of healthy protein, plus they are naturally rich in vitamin B12, iron, potassium, zinc, and selenium. This is the perfect meal for a hot summer evening when you don't feel like slaving over the stove. Preparing a big batch takes just a few minutes. Serve the mussels over spaghetti squash for a balanced meal.

Makes 6 to 8 (8- to 12-ounce) servings

4 pounds fresh, wild mussels

3 tablespoons coconut oil

1 cup diced shallots

6 cloves garlic, minced

½ cup chopped fresh parsley

1½ cups chicken or vegetable broth

1. Rinse the mussels thoroughly in cool water, picking through them to remove the beards. Discard any mussels that are broken or gaping open.

2. Heat the coconut oil in a large stockpot over medium heat. Add the shallots and garlic, and cook, uncovered, for 4 to 5 minutes, until softened. Add the mussels, then sprinkle with parsley and pour in the broth.

3. Increase the heat to high, cover the stockpot, and cook for 2 minutes. Remove the cover, stir once, replace the cover, and cook for another 3 to 4 minutes, until the mussels have opened.

4. To serve, spoon the mussels along with the broth into shallow bowls.

SEARED SCALLOPS
WITH BLUEBERRY GLAZE

This recipe, which stars tender seared scallops in a naturally sweet blueberry glaze, is the perfect blend of sweet and savory. Serve the scallops over mashed sweet potatoes or squash for a special-occasion meal. They also make an elegant appetizer served with toothpicks.

Makes 4 (4-ounce) servings

1 pound large wild sea scallops

1 cup fresh blueberries

¼ cup unsweetened apple juice

1 teaspoon grated fresh ginger

1 tablespoon pure maple syrup

1 tablespoon coconut oil

iodized salt and pepper

1. Rinse the scallops with cool water, and pat dry with paper towels.

2. To make the blueberry glaze, combine the blueberries, apple juice, ginger, and maple syrup in a small saucepan over medium heat. Gently mash the berries with a fork to break them up. Bring to a simmer, then reduce the heat to low, and cook for 10 minutes.

3. Heat the coconut oil in a large cast-iron skillet over medium heat. Season the scallops with salt and pepper, and add them to the skillet. Cook until lightly browned, about 3 minutes, then flip and cook for another 3 to 4 minutes, until browned and just cooked through.

4. Transfer to a serving platter. Spoon the blueberry glaze over the top to serve.

GINGER BEEF AND MUSHROOM STIR-FRY

Stir-fry is a go-to for many families because it is easy to prepare and to customize. This recipe features tender grass-fed beef flavored with fresh ginger and garlic.

Makes 4 to 6 (1½-cup) servings

1 cup beef broth

¼ cup white wine vinegar

1 tablespoon grated fresh ginger

2 cloves garlic, minced

1½ pounds grass-fed flank steak or sirloin

½ tablespoon coconut oil

2 cups chopped fresh broccoli florets

8 ounces cremini mushrooms, sliced

iodized salt and pepper

1. To make the marinade, whisk together the beef broth, white wine vinegar, ginger, and garlic in a small bowl. Set aside.

2. Season the steak with salt and pepper, then slice into strips. Place in a shallow dish, pour the marinade over the top, and turn to coat. Refrigerate for 20 to 30 minutes.

3. After the marinated steak has finished chilling, heat the coconut oil in a large skillet over medium-high heat. Add the steak strips, reserving the marinade, and cook for 3 to 4 minutes, turning halfway through. Cook until browned. Use a slotted spoon to transfer to a bowl, and reheat the skillet.

4. Add the broccoli, mushrooms, and reserved marinade. Stir-fry the vegetables for 4 to 5 minutes, until tender. Add the steak back to the skillet, and stir-fry for 1 minute or so, until heated through. Serve hot.

SPAGHETTI SQUASH
WITH GARLIC HERB MEATBALLS

These meatballs are full of flavor. The secret ingredient is grated zucchini, which helps to bulk up the meatballs while boosting their nutritional value. Serve the meatballs hot on a bed of baked spaghetti squash.

Makes 4 to 6 servings (serving size is ½ cup squash plus 3 meatballs)

1 cup finely grated zucchini

1 tablespoon agar-agar flakes

1 tablespoon warm water

1 pound grass-fed, lean ground beef

1 tablespoon chopped fresh parsley

1 tablespoon chopped fresh cilantro

1 tablespoon chopped fresh basil

2 cloves garlic, minced

1 small (3 to 4 pound) spaghetti squash

extra virgin olive oil, as needed

iodized salt and pepper

1. Preheat the oven to 400°F, and line a baking sheet with foil.

2. Spread the grated zucchini on a clean dish towel, roll it up, and wring out as much moisture as you can.

3. Whisk together the agar-agar flakes and warm water in a large bowl. Mix in the ground beef, grated zucchini, herbs, and garlic by hand. Season to taste with salt and pepper, and mix the ingredients together until thoroughly combined, taking care not to overmix.

4. Shape into 1½-inch balls by hand, and place on the baking sheet.

5. Cut the spaghetti squash in half, then scoop out and discard the seeds. Place the halves in a roasting pan cut side down, and add enough water to just cover the bottom. Roast for 30 to 45 minutes, until tender when pierced with a fork.

6. Add the meatballs to the oven after 10 minutes, and let cook for 25 to 30 minutes, until cooked through.

7. When the squash is tender, remove from the oven, and let cool for a few minutes until you can handle it. Remove the meatballs from the oven when cooked, and set aside. Use a fork to scoop out and shred the flesh of the squash into a bowl, then toss with enough olive oil to lightly coat the strands. Serve the squash topped with the meatballs.

HEARTY BEEF AND MUSHROOM STROGANOFF

This hot and hearty recipe features tender chunks of grass-fed beef simmered in a thick gravy with sliced mushrooms. Not only is this recipe sure to satiate your hunger, but it is the perfect dish to warm you up on a chilly evening.

Makes 4 to 6 (1½-cup) servings

2 tablespoons coconut oil

1½ pounds grass-fed sirloin beef, cut into strips

2 medium onions, sliced

2 cloves garlic, minced

1¼ cups beef broth, divided

1 (14-ounce) can coconut milk

8 ounces cremini mushrooms, thinly sliced

chopped fresh parsley

iodized salt and pepper

1. Heat the coconut oil in a large cast-iron skillet over medium-high heat. Season the beef with salt and pepper, and add it to the skillet. Cook for 1 to 2 minutes, until the underside is browned, then flip and cook for another minute. Use a slotted spoon to transfer to a bowl.

2. Reheat the skillet, and add the onions and garlic. Cook for 4 to 5 minutes, until the onions are translucent, stirring as needed.

3. Pour in ¼ cup of the beef broth, and stir to loosen the browned bits from the bottom of the skillet. Whisk in the coconut milk and remaining beef broth, and simmer until the mixture starts to thicken. Add the mushrooms, and return the beef to the skillet. Simmer for 5 to 8 minutes, until the mushrooms are tender and the sauce thickens.

4. Garnish with parsley to serve.

SEARED GINGER STEAK AND ONIONS

The combination of grated fresh ginger and coconut aminos, as a replacement for soy sauce, gives this seared ginger steak an Asian flavor. Serve the steak sliced over a green salad or pair it with your favorite steamed veggies.

Makes 4 (5- to 6-ounce) servings

½ cup beef broth

¼ cup coconut aminos

1 tablespoon extra virgin olive oil

1 tablespoon grated fresh ginger

2 cloves garlic, minced

2 (10–12-ounce) grass-fed sirloin steaks

1 tablespoon coconut oil

1 medium yellow onion, sliced

iodized salt and pepper

1. To make the marinade, whisk together the beef broth, coconut aminos, olive oil, ginger, and garlic in a small bowl. Season the steaks with salt and pepper, and place in a shallow dish. Pour the marinade over the steaks, and turn to coat. Cover the dish with plastic wrap, and chill in the refrigerator for at least 30 minutes.

2. Heat the coconut oil in a large skillet over medium-high heat. Add the onion, and cook for 4 to 5 minutes, until the onion is translucent. Push the onion to the edges of the skillet. Add the steaks, and cook for 3 to 4 minutes, until seared on the bottom. Flip and cook for another 3 to 4 minutes for medium-rare.

3. Remove the steaks to a cutting board, and let rest for 5 minutes. Slice the steaks into ¼-inch slices and serve topped with the browned onions.

LAMB STUFFED ACORN SQUASH

Acorn squash is loaded with vitamins A, B, and C, and folate. Enjoy this lamb-stuffed acorn squash as a main course or cut them in half to serve as a protein-packed side dish.

Makes 4 servings

2 acorn squash

1 teaspoon coconut oil

1 large yellow onion, chopped

2 cloves garlic, minced

1½ pounds grass-fed ground lamb

iodized salt and pepper

1. Preheat the oven to 400°F.

2. Cut each squash in half lengthwise, then scoop out the seeds and discard them. Place cut side down in a glass or ceramic baking dish. Add about ½ inch of water to the dish. Bake for 30 minutes, or until almost tender.

2. Meanwhile, melt the coconut oil in a large skillet over medium-high heat. Add the onion and garlic, and cook for 4 to 5 minutes, until softened. Stir in the ground lamb, and season with salt and pepper. Cook until the lamb is just browned, about 5 to 7 minutes.

3. Spoon the mixture into the squash halves. Place in the baking dish, and bake for about 10 minutes, until the squash is fork-tender.

LEMONGRASS VEAL LOLLIPOPS

A tasty twist on traditional kebabs, these veal "lollipops" are wrapped around fresh lemongrass stalks for a burst of flavor. In addition to being tender and full of protein, veal is rich in vitamin B12, iron, and zinc.

Makes 4 (2-lollipop) servings

8 fresh lemongrass stalks, cut to 8 inches long

8 grass-fed, boneless veal chops

¼ cup balsamic vinegar

1½ tablespoons extra virgin olive oil

1 tablespoon raw honey

1 teaspoon garlic powder

iodized salt and pepper

1. Preheat the grill to medium heat, and brush the grates with olive oil. If using a grill pan, spray with olive oil cooking spray and preheat to medium heat.

2. Trim the tops and root ends from the lemongrass, and set the stalks aside.

3. Lay the veal chops flat, and cover with plastic wrap. Pound with a flat meat mallet or the bottom of a heavy skillet until no thicker than ¼ inch. Season with salt and pepper. Wrap one piece of veal around each lemongrass stalk, and secure with a toothpick.

4. Whisk together the balsamic vinegar, olive oil, honey, and garlic powder in a small bowl. Brush the sauce over the veal lollipops, and place on the grill. Cook for 2 to 3 minutes on each side, brushing with sauce after turning. Transfer to a serving plate, and serve hot.

WHOLE ROASTED LEMON GARLIC CHICKEN

Roasting a chicken is a great way to feed a crowd, and this recipe for whole roasted lemon garlic chicken is surprisingly easy to prepare. Serve it with Oven-Roasted Acorn Squash (page 166) or a crunchy salad for a complete and satisfying meal.

Makes 8 servings

1 (5-pound) free-range, whole roaster chicken

¼ cup coconut oil

1 tablespoon fresh lemon juice

1 tablespoon minced fresh garlic

1 lemon, cut in half

2 sprigs fresh rosemary

2 sprigs fresh thyme

iodized salt and pepper

1. Preheat the oven to 450°F.

2. Remove the giblets from the chicken cavity, and set them aside. You can discard the giblets or cook them in the roasting pan next to the chicken. Rinse the chicken with cold water, inside and out, then pat dry with paper towels.

3. Melt the coconut oil in a small saucepan, and stir in the lemon juice and garlic.

4. Place the lemon halves, rosemary, and thyme in the chicken cavity then tie the legs of the chicken together with twine to keep them pressed against the body. Place the chicken in a roasting pan, breast side up.

5. Brush the coconut oil and garlic mixture liberally over the chicken, and season with salt and pepper.

6. Roast for 1 hour, basting with pan juices every 15 minutes. Check the internal temperature at the thickest part of the breast, and keep cooking if needed, until the temperature reaches 165°F.

7. Remove the chicken to a cutting board, and tent loosely with foil. Let rest for 10 minutes before carving to serve.

SWEET AND SOUR MANGO CHICKEN STIR-FRY

If you enjoy Chinese takeout, you will be a fan of this sweet and sour mango chicken stir-fry. A tasty (and healthy) twist on an old favorite, this dish gets most of its sweetness from the raw honey and fresh pineapple and mango.

Makes 4 to 6 (1½-cup) servings

½ cup unsweetened pineapple juice

¼ cup chicken broth

2 tablespoons apple cider vinegar

2 tablespoons raw honey

4 free-range, boneless, skinless chicken breasts

½ cup sifted coconut flour

¼ cup coconut oil, divided

1 medium yellow onion, chopped

1 medium red bell pepper, chopped

1 cup chopped fresh pineapple

1 cup chopped fresh mango

iodized salt and pepper

1. To make the sauce, whisk together the pineapple juice, chicken broth, apple cider vinegar, and honey in a small bowl. Set aside.

2. Cut the chicken breasts into bite-size pieces, and season with salt and pepper, then toss with the coconut flour in a large bowl.

3. Heat 2 tablespoons of the coconut oil in a large skillet over medium-high heat. Add the chicken, and cook until browned on all sides, about 5 to 7 minutes, then transfer to paper towels to drain.

4. Reheat the skillet with the remaining 2 tablespoons of coconut oil. Add the onion and bell pepper, and stir-fry for 3 to 4 minutes, until tender-crisp. Toss in the pineapple and mango chunks, then pour in the sauce. Bring the mixture to a simmer, and add the browned chicken. Remove when heated through, about 3 to 5 minutes. Serve immediately.

BRAISED CHICKEN WITH OLIVE TAPENADE

Braising is a cooking method that uses wet heat to preserve the natural flavor of the meat. This recipe yields a tender, juicy chicken leg topped with a homemade deliciously salty and tangy olive tapenade.

Makes 6 servings (serving size is 1 chicken leg plus 2 tablespoons tapenade)

FOR THE BRAISED CHICKEN

6 free-range, bone-in chicken legs, skin on

4 tablespoons extra virgin olive oil, divided, plus more as needed

3–4 cups chicken broth, divided

1 large sweet onion, chopped

2 small carrots, peeled and chopped

1 stalk celery, chopped

2 cloves garlic, minced

1 teaspoon chopped fresh oregano

iodized salt and pepper

FOR THE OLIVE TAPENADE

½ cup pitted and sliced black olives

½ cup pitted whole green olives

1 anchovy fillet, chopped

1 clove garlic, minced

½ teaspoon chopped fresh oregano

½ teaspoon chopped fresh thyme

2 tablespoons fresh lemon juice

1–2 tablespoons extra virgin olive oil

iodized salt

1. Preheat the oven to 450°F.

2. Season the chicken legs with salt and pepper. Heat 2 tablespoons of olive oil in a large ovenproof skillet over medium-high heat. Add the chicken to the skillet in a single layer, and cook until the chicken sizzles and the undersides are browned, about 5 minutes. Turn the chicken, and cook for 3 to 5 minutes on the other side, until browned. Transfer to a plate.

3. Reheat the skillet, adding more oil if needed. Stir in 1 cup of chicken broth, scraping any browned bits from the bottom of the skillet. Simmer for 1 to 2 minutes, then pour the pan liquid into a small bowl and set aside.

4. Reheat the skillet with the remaining 2 tablespoons of olive oil, and add the onion, carrots, and celery. Season with salt and pepper to taste, and cook for 8 to 10 minutes, stirring as needed, until the vegetables are tender. Stir in the garlic and oregano, then add the chicken legs back to the skillet. Pour in the reserved pan liquid, and add enough of the remaining broth to come about halfway up the thickness of the chicken legs. Bring the liquid to a simmer, then place the skillet in the oven.

5. Bake for 5 minutes, then reduce the heat to 325°F, and cook for 35 to 40 minutes, until the internal temperature of the chicken reaches 165°F.

6. While the chicken is cooking, prepare the tapenade by combining the black and green olives in a food processor. Pulse until finely chopped, then add the anchovy, garlic, oregano, thyme, and lemon juice. Season with salt to taste, and pulse until finely chopped. While pulsing, drizzle in the olive oil until the desired consistency is reached.

7. During the last 10 minutes the chicken is in the oven, spread 1 to 2 tablespoons of the olive tapenade on each chicken leg. When the chicken is cooked, transfer to a large platter. Cover loosely with foil, and let rest for 5 to 10 minutes before serving.

MAPLE LIME CHICKEN DRUMSTICKS

Marinated in a maple lime sauce, these chicken drumsticks are juicy and tender in the middle with a sweet, crispy skin. This is the perfect meal to break in your grill after a long winter, but you can also prepare it on the stovetop with a grill pan or using the broiler in your oven set to medium heat. The sweetness of these chicken drumsticks would contrast well with a savory side dish like Garlic Sautéed Spinach (page 171).

Makes 4 to 6 (2- to 3-drumstick) servings

12 free-range chicken drumsticks, skin on

½ cup pure maple syrup

½ cup fresh lime juice

¼ cup apple cider vinegar

1 tablespoon fresh lime zest

1 clove garlic, minced

extra virgin olive oil, as needed

1. Place the chicken in a large zip-top plastic freezer bag.

2. To make the marinade, whisk together the maple syrup, lime juice, apple cider vinegar, lime zest, and garlic in a medium bowl. Pour into the freezer bag, and shake to coat the chicken. Chill in the refrigerator for at least 4 hours.

3. Preheat the grill to high heat (about 400°F), and brush the grates with olive oil. If preparing this recipe on the stovetop, grease a grill pan with olive oil cooking spray and preheat to high heat.

4. Remove the chicken from the bag, reserving the liquid, and place on the grill. Cook for 20 to 25 minutes, turning every 5 minutes or so, until cooked through.

5. Meanwhile, pour the reserved marinade into a small saucepan, and bring to a simmer over medium heat. Cook the sauce for 10 to 15 minutes, until thickened. Serve the chicken hot, and drizzle with the maple lime sauce.

GUACAMOLE STUFFED TURKEY BREAST

These tender baked turkey breasts become infused with the flavor of fresh avocado which also helps to keep the meat moist during cooking. In addition to adding a rich flavor to this dish, ripe avocado is a natural source of healthy monounsaturated fats while turkey provides lean protein, B vitamins, selenium, and zinc.

Makes 4 (6-ounce) servings with ¼ cup guacamole each

FOR THE GUACAMOLE

1 large ripe avocado

3 tablespoons diced red onion

1 teaspoon fresh lime juice

1 clove garlic, minced

½ teaspoon iodized salt

FOR THE TURKEY

1½ pounds free-range, boneless, skinless turkey breast

1 tablespoon coconut oil

iodized salt and pepper

1. Preheat the oven to 400°F, and spray a baking dish with olive oil cooking spray.

2. To prepare the guacamole, spoon the avocado flesh into a medium bowl, and mash well with a fork. Stir in the red onion, lime juice, garlic, and salt until well combined.

3. Cut the turkey breast into four even pieces and lay them flat on a cutting board. Cover with plastic wrap, and pound with a flat meat mallet to about ½ inch thick.

4. Divide the guacamole evenly among the four pieces of turkey, spreading it over the entire piece. Roll up the pieces of turkey, and secure them with kitchen string.

5. Heat the coconut oil in a large skillet over medium-high heat. Season the turkey rolls with salt and pepper. Place in the skillet, and cook for 1 to 2 minutes until browned. Flip and cook until browned on the other side, then transfer to the baking dish.

6. Bake for 25 to 30 minutes, until cooked through. Let rest for about 5 minutes before serving.

GARLIC HERB ROASTED PORK TENDERLOIN

Boneless pork tenderloins are flavored with fresh garlic, roasted until tender with a crispy herb crust. This recipe is easy to multiply, and you can customize it with fresh herbs plucked from your garden. Serve this roasted pork tenderloin with Balsamic Roasted Beets (page 159), or Honey Dill Baby Carrots (page 163) for a balanced meal.

Makes 4 to 6 (4- to 8-ounce) servings

2 (1–1½ pound) grass-fed boneless pork tenderloins

2 tablespoons chopped fresh rosemary

1 tablespoon chopped fresh oregano

1 tablespoon chopped fresh thyme

6 cloves garlic, minced

¼ cup extra virgin olive oil

iodized salt and pepper

1. Preheat the oven to 375°F, and line a rimmed baking sheet with foil.

2. Season the tenderloins with salt and pepper, and place on the baking sheet.

3. Place the rosemary, oregano, thyme, and garlic in a food processor. Pulse several times to chop, then drizzle in the oil while the processor runs. Blend into a smooth paste, then spread over the tenderloins.

4. Roast for 10 minutes. Flip the tenderloins, then roast for another 8 to 10 minutes, until the internal temperature reaches 155°F.

5. Remove to a cutting board, and cover loosely with foil. Let rest for 10 minutes before slicing to serve.

BACON WRAPPED PORK MEDALLIONS

Pork medallions are wrapped in bacon and grilled until the bacon is crisp then drizzled with a sweet maple glaze. Grass-fed pork is loaded with lean protein as well as a number of important B vitamins, making this meaty dish a natural source of zinc, a mineral known to support immune system health.

Makes 4 (2-medallion) servings

1 (1½–2 pound) grass-fed boneless pork tenderloin

8 slices uncured bacon

¼ cup balsamic vinegar

2 tablespoons pure maple syrup

½ teaspoon garlic powder

iodized salt and pepper

1. Preheat the grill to medium-high heat, and brush the grates with olive oil. To prepare on the stovetop, spray a grill pan with olive oil cooking spray and preheat to medium-high heat.

2. Season the pork tenderloins with salt and pepper then cut them into 8 medallions, each about the width of a piece of bacon. Wrap each medallion in bacon, and thread them onto metal skewers.

3. Grill the medallions for 6 to 8 minutes on each side, until almost cooked through.

4. Meanwhile, whisk together the balsamic vinegar, maple syrup, and garlic powder in a small bowl. Brush the glaze on the medallions, and cook for 1 minute more on each side. Serve hot.

APPLE CRANBERRY STUFFED PORK LOIN

Dress up a plain pork tenderloin with tart apple and tender cranberries. Apples are loaded with antioxidants and flavonoids while cranberries provide plenty of vitamin C, manganese, and dietary fiber to support healthy digestion.

Makes 4 servings

1 (1½–2 pound) grass-fed boneless pork tenderloin

1 medium tart apple, diced

1 cup finely chopped mushrooms

½ cup chopped unsweetened dried cranberries

¼ cup diced white onion

1 clove garlic, minced

2 tablespoons pure maple syrup

iodized salt and pepper

1. Preheat the oven to 375°F.

2. Lay the tenderloin on a cutting board, and use a sharp knife to slice down the middle, halfway through the thickness of the meat. Unfold the tenderloin, and lay it flat. Place two or three pieces of plastic wrap over it, and gently pound with a flat meat mallet until about ½ inch thick.

3. To make the stuffing, combine the apple, mushrooms, cranberries, onion, and garlic in a medium bowl. Add the maple syrup, and season with salt and pepper to taste. Stir until well combined.

4. Spoon the stuffing lengthwise down the middle of the tenderloin, leaving a 1-inch border all the way around. Roll up tightly, and secure with kitchen string. Place in a roasting pan.

5. Roast for 1 hour, or until the internal temperature of the meat reaches 145°F. Transfer to a cutting board, and let rest for 5 minutes before slicing to serve.

CHAPTER 9
Vegan and Vegetarian Dishes

VEGETABLE STUFFED ZUCCHINI BOATS

Warm, tender zucchini stuffed with a vegetable medley makes for an exquisite vegan meal. Roasting the zucchini in olive oil before stuffing it with the herbed vegetable medley makes this dish fragrant and flavorful.

Makes 4 servings

2 medium zucchini

extra virgin olive oil, as needed

1 teaspoon coconut oil

1 medium yellow onion, diced

1 cup diced mushrooms

2 cups chopped beet greens

2 cloves garlic, minced

1 teaspoon dried oregano

½ teaspoon dried basil

iodized salt and pepper

1. Preheat the oven to 375°F.

2. Trim the ends of the zucchini, then cut in half lengthwise. Use a spoon to scoop out the flesh, leaving a ¼-inch border all around. Brush the cut sides of the zucchini with olive oil, and season lightly with salt and pepper. Place cut side up in a glass or ceramic baking dish, and bake for 15 minutes.

3. Meanwhile, heat the coconut oil in a medium skillet over medium-high heat. Add the onion, and cook until translucent, about 4 to 5 minutes. Stir in the mushrooms, beet greens, and garlic, and season with salt and pepper to taste. Cook for 3 to 4 minutes until the beet greens are wilted, then stir in the oregano and basil.

4. Spoon the vegetable filling into the zucchini halves. Bake for another 20 to 30 minutes, until the zucchini is very tender.

SAUTÉED SPAGHETTI SQUASH WITH VEGGIES

Spaghetti squash makes a tasty alternative to pasta because it's satisfying and filling—and the cooked flesh, scraped out of the shell, even looks like angel hair pasta. This winter squash is rich in vitamins A and C, and an excellent source of dietary fiber, manganese, potassium, and magnesium. This recipe goes well with lighter entrees like Rosemary Citrus Swordfish Steaks or you can enjoy it on its own as a vegan dinner option.

Makes 6 to 8 (½-cup) servings

1 large (6 to 7 pound) spaghetti squash

extra virgin olive oil, as needed

1 tablespoon coconut oil

1 medium yellow onion, chopped

2 cloves garlic, minced

1 small zucchini, peeled and diced

1½ cups diced white mushrooms

iodized salt and pepper

1. Preheat the oven to 400°F, and line a rimmed baking sheet with foil.

2. Cut the spaghetti squash in half lengthwise, then scoop out and discard the seeds. Brush the cut sides with olive oil, and season with salt and pepper. Place the halves cut side down on the baking sheet. Roast for about 20 minutes, until the squash can be pierced easily with a knife.

3. Meanwhile, melt the coconut oil in a large skillet over medium-high heat. Add the onion and garlic, and cook for 5 to 6 minutes, until tender. Stir in the zucchini and mushrooms, and cook for 4 to 5 minutes, until tender.

4. Remove the squash from the oven, and let sit until cool enough to handle. Shred the flesh with a fork, scoop into a large bowl, and toss with the sautéed veggies.

5. Adjust the seasoning to taste, and serve hot.

BALSAMIC ROASTED VEGETABLE FLATBREAD

Tender vegetables roasted with a balsamic marinade are spread atop a warm coconut flour flatbread in this dish. Feel free to use whatever vegetables you have on hand to customize this recipe to your taste, and don't be afraid to garnish the flatbread with fresh herbs for a beautiful and aromatic presentation.

Makes 4 servings

FOR THE VEGETABLES

1 medium zucchini, diced

1 small yellow onion, thinly sliced

8 ounces cremini mushrooms, thinly sliced

2 cloves garlic, thinly sliced

2 tablespoons extra virgin olive oil

2 tablespoons balsamic vinegar

iodized salt and pepper

FOR THE FLATBREAD

½ cup sifted coconut flour

½ teaspoon baking powder

½ teaspoon baking soda

½ teaspoon iodized salt

¼ cup plus 2 tablespoons agar-agar flakes

¾ cup warm water

½ cup canned coconut milk

extra virgin olive oil, as needed

1. Preheat the oven to 425°F, and line a rimmed baking sheet with foil and another baking sheet with parchment paper.

2. Combine the zucchini, onion, mushrooms, and garlic in a large bowl. Toss with the olive oil and balsamic vinegar, then season with salt and pepper to taste. Spread on the foil-lined baking sheet, and bake for 15 to 20 minutes, until tender, then remove from the oven to cool slightly.

3. Meanwhile, make the flatbread batter by whisking together the coconut flour, baking powder, baking soda, and salt in a large bowl. In a medium bowl, whisk together the agar-agar flakes and warm water. Whisk the agar-agar mixture and the coconut milk into the dry ingredients until smooth.

4. To cook the flatbread, spray an 8-inch skillet with olive oil cooking spray and preheat over medium heat. Spread about a quarter of the batter in the skillet, and cook for 1 to 2 minutes, until firm. Carefully flip the flatbread, and cook for another 1 to 2 minutes, until firm and lightly browned.

5. Transfer to the parchment-lined baking sheet, and repeat with the remaining batter. Once all four flatbreads are cooked, brush the tops with olive oil, and preheat the broiler in your oven to high heat.

6. Spoon the roasted vegetables over the flatbreads, and broil for 1 to 2 minutes, until heated through. Serve warm.

GARLIC HERB FLATBREAD WITH FRESH PESTO

Warm flatbread flavored with garlic and herbs makes a perfect vehicle for fresh basil pesto. Although pesto is traditionally made with pine nuts and Parmesan cheese, this recipe is dairy-free and nut-free in keeping with the Hashimoto's diet plan.

Makes 4 servings

FOR THE PESTO

2 cups chopped fresh basil

½ cup unsweetened shredded coconut

1 tablespoon fresh lemon juice

1 clove garlic, minced

3–4 tablespoons extra virgin olive oil

iodized salt

FOR THE FLATBREAD

½ cup sifted coconut flour

½ teaspoon baking powder

½ teaspoon baking soda

½ teaspoon iodized salt

¼ teaspoon dried rosemary

¼ teaspoon dried oregano

2 cloves garlic, minced

6 tablespoons agar-agar flakes

¾ cup warm water

½ cup canned coconut milk

1. To make the pesto, combine the basil, coconut, lemon juice, and garlic in a food processor. Blend well. With the processor running, drizzle in the olive oil until the pesto reaches the desired consistency. Season with salt to taste, and set aside.

2. To make the flatbread batter, whisk together the coconut flour, baking powder, baking soda, salt, rosemary, oregano, and garlic in a large bowl. In a medium bowl, whisk together the agar-agar flakes and warm water. Whisk the agar-agar mixture and the coconut milk into the dry ingredients until smooth.

3. To cook the flatbread, spray an 8-inch skillet with olive oil cooking spray and preheat over medium heat. Spread about a quarter of the batter in the skillet, and cook for 1 to 2 minutes, until firm. Carefully flip the flatbread, and cook for another 1 to 2 minutes, until firm and lightly browned. Remove the

flatbread to a plate and cover with foil to keep warm. Repeat with the remaining batter.

4. Once all four flatbreads are cooked, spread with the pesto and serve.

ROSEMARY FLATBREAD WITH OLIVE TAPENADE

Fresh rosemary baked into a tender flatbread is absolutely perfect when topped with homemade olive tapenade. Inspired by the flavors of the Mediterranean region, this recipe is a great way to shake up your dietary routine. For a complete meal, serve with soup or salad.

Makes 4 servings (serving size is 1 flatbread plus ¼ cup tapenade)

FOR THE TAPENADE

1 cup pitted black olives

1 cup pitted green olives

2 tablespoons drained capers

1 clove garlic, minced

1 tablespoon chopped fresh basil

1 tablespoon chopped fresh parsley

1 teaspoon chopped fresh thyme

1 teaspoon chopped fresh oregano

3–4 tablespoons extra virgin olive oil

iodized salt and pepper

FOR THE FLATBREAD

½ cup sifted coconut flour

½ teaspoon baking powder

½ teaspoon baking soda

¼ cup plus 2 tablespoons agar-agar flakes

¾ cup warm water

½ cup canned coconut milk

2 tablespoons chopped fresh rosemary

chopped fresh parsley

1. To make the tapenade, combine the olives, capers, and garlic in a food processor. Pulse to chop, then add the basil, parsley, thyme, and oregano. Drizzle in the olive oil while pulsing the mixture until finely chopped. Season with salt and pepper to taste.

2. To make the flatbread batter, combine the coconut flour, baking powder, baking soda, and salt in a large bowl. In a medium bowl, whisk together the agar-agar flakes and warm water. Whisk the agar-agar mixture, coconut milk, and rosemary into the dry ingredients until smooth.

3. To cook the flatbread, spray an 8-inch skillet with olive oil cooking spray and preheat over medium heat. Spread about a quarter of the batter in the skillet, and cook for 1 to 2 minutes, until firm. Carefully flip the flatbread, and cook for another 1 to 2 minutes, until firm and lightly browned.

4. Transfer to a plate and wrap with foil to keep warm, and repeat with the remaining batter. Once all four flatbreads are cooked, spoon the olive tapenade over them. Garnish with parsley to serve.

HEARTY MUSHROOM PIE WITH COCONUT FLOUR CRUST

Tender chunks of mushroom baked into a creamy vegetable sauce makes a hearty filling for a fresh coconut flour pie crust. A tasty vegan alternative to chicken pot pie, this recipe is surprisingly easy to prepare and will feed the whole family.

Makes 4 to 6 servings

FOR THE CRUST

2 tablespoons agar-agar flakes

2 tablespoons warm water

½ cup melted coconut oil

1 tablespoon agave

¼ teaspoon iodized salt

¾ cup sifted coconut flour

FOR THE FILLING

2 tablespoons grass-fed ghee

1 medium yellow onion, diced

2 medium carrots, peeled and diced

2 stalks celery, diced

8 ounces mushrooms, diced

1 clove garlic, minced

½ teaspoon dried oregano

¼ teaspoon dried thyme

¼ cup arrowroot powder

1½ cups vegetable broth

iodized salt and pepper

1. Preheat the oven to 400°F.

2. To make the crust, whisk together the agar-agar flakes and warm water in a medium bowl. Add the coconut oil, agave, and salt, and whisk until smooth. Whisk in the coconut flour, and stir until the mixture forms a dough that holds together well. Gather by hand into a ball, and press into the bottom and sides of a 9-inch glass pie plate. Prick the bottom and sides of the crust with a fork. Bake for 6 to 8 minutes until the crust is firm, then remove, and set aside while you prepare the filling.

3. To make the filling, melt the ghee in a medium saucepan over medium heat. Add the onion, carrots, celery, and mushrooms, then season with salt and pepper to taste. Cook until the vegetables are tender, then stir in the garlic, oregano, and thyme. Whisk the arrowroot powder into the vegetable broth,

and drizzle the mixture into the saucepan while stirring. Simmer for 10 to 12 minutes, until thick and hot. Pour into the prepared crust.

4. Bake for 8 to 10 minutes, until the crust is browned.

EASY ZUCCHINI GARLIC BISQUE

Although light in flavor, zucchini is packed with powerful nutrients like dietary fiber, vitamin C, folate, and beta-carotene. In this recipe, it combines with the vegetable broth to make a subtle and elegant, creamy bisque. You can substitute other summer squashes for the zucchini, if desired.

Makes 4 to 6 (1-cup) servings

3 pounds zucchini, chopped

2 medium sweet onions, chopped

2 tablespoons minced garlic

2–3 tablespoons extra virgin olive oil

8 cups vegetable broth

½ cup chopped fresh basil

1½ teaspoons dried oregano

iodized salt and pepper

1. Preheat the oven to 375°F, and line a rimmed baking sheet with foil.

2. Toss together the zucchini, onions, and garlic with the olive oil, and spread the mixture on the baking sheet. Season with salt and pepper to taste. Bake until tender, for 30 to 35 minutes, turning once halfway through.

3. Heat the vegetable broth in a large saucepan over medium-high heat. Add the cooked vegetables, and bring to a simmer. Stir in the basil and oregano, then puree the soup with an immersion blender. Adjust the seasoning to taste. Serve hot.

HEARTY WINTER VEGETABLE SOUP

If you are looking for the perfect recipe to clean out your vegetable drawer, give this hearty soup a try. The beauty of this recipe is that it can be made with just about any vegetables you happen to have on hand, so feel free to get creative.

Makes 4 to 6 (1-cup) servings

1 tablespoon coconut oil

1 medium yellow onion, chopped

2 cloves garlic, minced

1 (3-pound) sugar pumpkin, peeled, seeded, and chopped

2 medium carrots, peeled and chopped

2 medium parsnips, peeled and chopped

1 cup chopped fresh butternut squash

6 cups vegetable broth

½ teaspoon ground cinnamon

iodized salt and pepper

1. Melt the coconut oil in a large saucepan over medium-high heat. Add the onion and garlic. Cook until the onion is translucent, about 4 to 5 minutes. Stir in the pumpkin, carrots, parsnips, and butternut squash. Add the vegetable broth, cinnamon, and salt and pepper to taste. Bring to a boil, then reduce the heat and simmer for 25 to 30 minutes, until the vegetables are very tender.

2. Puree the soup with an immersion blender. Adjust the seasoning to taste. Serve hot.

CREAMY LEEK AND MUSHROOM SOUP

This leek and mushroom soup has a rich, earthy flavor, and the addition of coconut milk makes it creamy without making it too heavy. Leeks are a member of the onion family and they are rich in flavonoids and antioxidants. Fresh leeks can help to provide cardiovascular support, and their polyphenol content offers natural anti-inflammatory benefits as well.

Makes 6 (1-cup) servings

1 tablespoon coconut oil

1 medium sweet onion, diced

2 small leeks, chopped (white and light green parts only)

1 tablespoon minced garlic

2 teaspoons chopped fresh tarragon

2 pounds fresh white mushrooms (or mushrooms of your choice), sliced

4 cups vegetable broth

1 cup canned coconut milk

iodized salt and pepper

1. Heat the coconut oil in a large stockpot over medium heat. Add the onion and leeks, stirring to coat with oil, and cook for 6 to 8 minutes, until soft. Stir in the garlic and tarragon, then cook for 1 minute, until fragrant. Add the mushrooms, and cook for 4 to 5 minutes, until the liquid has cooked off. Stir in the vegetable broth and coconut milk, and season with salt and pepper to taste. Reduce the heat and simmer for about 5 minutes, then remove from the heat.

2. Puree the soup with an immersion blender, and adjust the seasoning to taste. Serve hot.

GINGER GRILLED ZUCCHINI STEAKS

Marinated in a fresh ginger dressing, these grilled zucchini steaks are the perfect way to prepare fresh zucchini because grilling brings out the tenderness of the vegetable. The zucchini contributes dietary fiber, while the fresh ginger adds natural anti-inflammatory and analgesic benefits. Serve with a light vegetable salad for a complete meal.

Makes 4 to 6 (2-slice) servings

½ cup coconut aminos	1 tablespoon grated fresh ginger
½ cup vegetable broth	2 cloves garlic, minced
¼ cup extra virgin olive oil	2–3 pounds zucchini
1 tablespoon agave	iodized salt and pepper

1. To make the marinade, whisk together the coconut aminos, vegetable broth, olive oil, agave, ginger, and garlic in a medium bowl.

2. Cut the zucchini in half width-wise, then slice lengthwise into ½-inch thick slices. Place the zucchini slices in a shallow dish in a single layer, and pour the ginger marinade over them. Season with salt and pepper to taste. Turn the slices to coat, and let soak at room temperature for about 30 minutes.

3. Preheat the grill to medium-high heat, and brush the grates with olive oil. If using the stovetop, grease a grill pan with olive oil cooking spray and preheat over medium-high heat. Place the zucchini slices on the grill, and cook for about 5 minutes. Carefully flip the zucchini, and cook for another 3 to 5 minutes, until tender. Serve hot.

ROASTED VEGETABLE CREPES

Warm coconut flour crepes layered with pureed roasted vegetables makes for a simple but satisfying meal. The key to perfect crepes is to avoid overcooking them. They should be warm and pliable, and just barely browned on both sides.

Makes 4 to 6 servings (serving size is 2 crepes plus ½ cup vegetables)

FOR THE VEGETABLES

1 medium zucchini, halved lengthwise and diced

2 large carrots, peeled and diced

1 medium beet, peeled and diced

1 large yellow onion, diced

8 ounces cremini mushrooms, chopped

3 cloves garlic, thinly sliced

2–3 tablespoons extra virgin olive oil

up to 1 cup vegetable broth

iodized salt and pepper

FOR THE CREPES

1 cup agar-agar flakes

1 cup warm water

¾ cup canned coconut milk

1 teaspoon fresh lemon juice

½ cup sifted coconut flour

¼ teaspoon baking soda

pinch of iodized salt

1. Preheat the oven to 425°F, and line a rimmed baking sheet with parchment paper.

2. Toss together the zucchini, carrots, beet, onion, mushrooms, and garlic with the olive oil. Spread on the baking sheet, and season with salt and pepper to taste. Roast for 25 to 35 minutes, until very tender.

3. Transfer the cooked vegetables to a food processor. Add vegetable broth as needed, and blend into a thick puree. Transfer to a covered saucepan over low heat to keep warm.

4. To make the crepe batter, whisk together the agar-agar flakes and water in a medium bowl. In a separate medium bowl, whisk together the coconut milk and lemon juice, and let rest

for 5 minutes. Combine the coconut flour, baking soda, and salt in a large bowl, then slowly whisk in the agar-agar mixture and the coconut milk mixture until smooth. Let the batter sit for 10 minutes to thicken.

5. To cook the crepes, preheat an 8-inch skillet over medium-low heat, and spray with olive oil cooking spray. Spoon about ¼ cup of crepe batter into the skillet, and tilt to coat the bottom. Cook until the center is set, about 1 minutes, then carefully flip the crepe. Cook for another 30 to 60 seconds, until set. Remove to a plate, and cover with foil to keep warm until ready to assemble. Repeat with the remaining batter until all the crepes are cooked.

6. Lay the crepes flat, and spoon about ¼ cup of the vegetable puree down the middle of each. Fold or roll up the crepes to serve.

CREAMY MUSHROOM GREEN ONION CREPES

Slices of fresh mushroom and scallions tossed in a creamy coconut sauce makes for an indulgent and hearty crepe filling. Serve these crepes for breakfast or dinner—they are sure to be a hit any time of day.

Makes 6 to 8 (2-crepe) servings

FOR THE CREPES

¾ cup canned coconut milk

½ teaspoon fresh lemon juice

1 cup agar-agar flakes

1 cup warm water

½ cup sifted coconut flour

¼ teaspoon baking soda

¼ teaspoon iodized salt

FOR THE FILLING

1 teaspoon coconut oil

8 ounces cremini mushrooms, thinly sliced

1 (14-ounce) can coconut milk

¼ cup warm water

2–3 tablespoons arrowroot powder

1 bunch green onions, white and green parts, thinly sliced

iodized salt and pepper

1. To make the crepe batter, whisk together the coconut milk and lemon juice in a medium bowl, and let rest for 5 minutes. Sprinkle the agar-agar flakes over the mixture, then whisk in the warm water. In a large bowl, combine the coconut flour, baking soda, and salt. Whisk the wet ingredients into the dry until smooth. Let rest 10 minutes.

2. To make the filling, melt the coconut oil in a medium skillet over medium heat. Add the mushrooms, and cook until the liquid has evaporated, about 5 to 6 minutes. Stir in the coconut milk, and season with salt and pepper to taste. Whisk together the water and arrowroot powder, then whisk the mixture into the skillet. Cook until thickened, about 5 minutes, then turn off the heat and cover to keep warm.

3. To cook the crepes, heat an 8-inch skillet over medium-low heat, and spray with olive oil cooking spray. Spoon about ¼ cup of batter into the skillet, and tilt to coat the bottom. Cook until the center is set, about 1 minute, then carefully flip the crepe. Cook for another 30 to 60 seconds, until set. The cooked crepes should be pliable and just brown. Remove to a plate and cover with foil to keep warm. Repeat with the remaining batter until all the crepes are cooked.

4. Lay the crepes flat, and spoon about ¼ cup of the mushroom mixture down the middle of each. Fold or roll the crepes, and top with more of the mushroom mixture. Garnish with green onions to serve.

SWEET POTATO WAFFLES WITH CINNAMON COCONUT CREAM

If you are feeling indulgent, enjoy these waffles as breakfast for dinner. The waffles are crisp on the outside, tender in the middle, and topped with lightly sweetened cinnamon coconut cream.

Makes 4 to 6 servings (serving is 1 waffle plus 2 tablespoons cream)

FOR THE CINNAMON COCONUT CREAM

1 (14-ounce) can coconut milk, refrigerated overnight

1–2 tablespoons agave

½ teaspoon ground cinnamon

FOR THE WAFFLES

3 tablespoons agar-agar flakes

3 tablespoons warm water

1½ pounds sweet potatoes, peeled and grated

2 tablespoons melted coconut oil

½–1 teaspoon ground cinnamon

1. To make the cinnamon coconut cream, open the can of coconut milk from the bottom, and spoon the solids into a medium bowl. Discard the liquid or save it for another recipe. Add the agave and cinnamon, then blend with a hand mixer until thick and creamy, about 3 to 5 minutes.

2. Preheat your waffle iron, and spray with olive oil cooking spray.

3. Meanwhile, make the waffle batter by whisking together the agar-agar flakes and water in a large bowl. Stir in the grated sweet potato, coconut oil, and cinnamon until well combined in a thick batter.

4. Spoon ¼ to ½ cup of batter into the preheated waffle iron. Cook until just browned and crisp on the edges. Transfer to a plate, and cover with foil to keep warm. Repeat with the remaining batter.

5. Serve warm with a dollop of cinnamon coconut cream.

GOITROGEN ALERT: max 6 to 8 servings per week

BALSAMIC GRILLED PORTOBELLO CAPS

Marinated in balsamic vinegar and grilled, these tender portobello mushroom caps are a satiating addition atop a fresh green salad. They can also be enjoyed as an entree paired with your favorite vegan or vegetarian side dish.

Makes 6 servings

¾ cup extra virgin olive oil

¼ cup plus 2 tablespoons balsamic vinegar

1 tablespoon agave

1 tablespoon minced garlic

½ teaspoon iodized salt

6 large portobello mushroom caps

1. Make the marinade by whisking together the olive oil, balsamic vinegar, agave, garlic, and salt in a medium bowl.

2. Remove the stems from the mushroom caps and save them for another recipe, then place the caps in a shallow dish. Pour the marinade over the top, turning to coat. Let soak for 15 minutes at room temperature.

3. Preheat your grill to medium-high heat, and brush the grates with olive oil. If preparing on the stovetop, grease a grill pan with olive oil cooking spray and preheat to medium-high heat. Place the mushroom caps on the grill, underside up, and cook for 4 minutes. Flip the mushrooms, and cook for another 3 to 4 minutes, until tender. Serve hot.

HERB ROASTED VEGETABLE MEDLEY

This recipe gathers some favorite vegetables into one dish packed with dietary fiber and healthy nutrients. Fresh herbs and garlic add tons of flavor. But don't feel you have to follow the recipe exactly—you can use whatever vegetables you have on hand.

Makes 4 to 6 (1½-cup) servings

1 tablespoon coconut oil

1 large yellow onion, chopped

½ inch grated fresh ginger

2 cloves garlic, minced

1 pound sweet potatoes, peeled and chopped

½ pound fresh baby carrots

2 medium parsnips, peeled and thickly sliced

1 medium zucchini, sliced into ½-inch rounds

1 cup chopped fresh butternut squash

¼ cup extra virgin olive oil

1 tablespoon chopped fresh rosemary

2 teaspoons chopped fresh thyme

2 teaspoons chopped fresh oregano

iodized salt and pepper

1. Preheat the oven to 400°F and line a rimmed baking sheet with parchment paper.

2. Melt the coconut oil in a large skillet over medium-high heat. Add the onion, and cook for 4 to 5 minutes, until tender, then stir in the ginger and garlic. Cook for 1 minute, until fragrant, then spoon the mixture into a large bowl. Add the sweet potatoes, carrots, parsnips, zucchini, and butternut squash. Drizzle with the olive oil, and toss with the rosemary, thyme, and oregano. Season with salt and pepper to taste.

3. Spread the mixture on the prepared baking sheet and roast for 20 minutes, then stir the vegetables and roast for another 15 to 20 minutes, until tender.

COCONUT MIXED VEGETABLE CURRY

Tender vegetables in a creamy coconut curry, this dish is as fragrant and delicious as it is wholesome and nutritious. Curry powder contains the active ingredient curcumin, which is a powerful antioxidant as well as a strong anti-inflammatory.

Makes 3 to 4 (1½-cup) servings

1 tablespoon coconut oil

1 large yellow onion, chopped

2 cloves garlic, minced

1 (14-ounce) can coconut milk

2 tablespoons curry powder

1 tablespoon agave

1 medium sweet potato, peeled and chopped

2 medium carrots, peeled and chopped

8 ounces mushrooms, thinly sliced

4 ounces fresh green beans, ends trimmed

fresh cilantro leaves

iodized salt

1. Melt the coconut oil in a deep skillet over medium-high heat. Add the onion and garlic, and cook until the onion is translucent, about 4 to 5 minutes.

2. Stir in the coconut milk, curry powder, and agave. Season with salt to taste. Add the sweet potato and carrots, then cover and cook on low heat for 5 minutes.

3. Stir in the mushrooms and green beans, and simmer uncovered for 3 to 5 minutes, until heated through. Turn up the heat for a few minutes, if needed, to thicken the sauce.

4. Serve hot. Spoon the curry into individual bowls, and garnish with cilantro leaves.

LEMON ARTICHOKE ZUCCHINI "PASTA"

Just because traditional wheat pasta is not included in the Hashimoto's diet doesn't mean you can't enjoy noodles. These noodles are made from fresh zucchini and tossed with roasted artichokes, fresh lemon juice, and garlic for a flavorful and healthy dish.

Makes 4 (1½-cup) servings

2½ pounds fresh zucchini

1 tablespoon coconut oil

1 (14-ounce) can artichoke hearts, drained and chopped

2 cloves garlic, minced

1 tablespoon extra virgin olive oil

2–3 tablespoons fresh lemon juice

iodized salt and pepper

1. Use a spiralizer or vegetable peeler to peel the zucchini into noodle-like ribbons.

2. Heat the coconut oil in a large skillet over medium heat then add the chopped artichoke hearts and cook for 3 to 4 minutes.

3. Stir in the garlic and cook for 1 to 2 minutes, then add in the olive oil and zucchini noodles, then sauté for 2 to 3 minutes until heated through.

4. Remove from the stovetop and drizzle with lemon juice, and season with salt and pepper to taste and serve hot.

CREAMY LEMON GARLIC ZUCCHINI "PASTA"

For a simple but satisfying meal, whip up a batch of this "pasta" made from zucchini and coated with a creamy lemon garlic sauce. The sauce has the perfect combination of tangy citrus and fresh garlic flavors, and the noodles take only a few minutes to cook.

Makes 4 to 6 (1½-cup) servings

5 pounds zucchini

2 (14-ounce) cans coconut milk

juice and zest of 1 lemon

1 tablespoon minced garlic

3–4 tablespoons fresh chopped parsley

1 tablespoon coconut oil

iodized salt and pepper

1. Use a spiralizer or vegetable peeler to peel the zucchini into noodle-like ribbons.

2. To make the sauce, spoon the coconut milk into a small saucepan over medium heat. Whisk in the lemon juice, lemon zest, garlic, and parsley. Season with salt and pepper to taste, and bring to a simmer while you prepare the zucchini pasta.

3. Melt the coconut oil in a deep skillet over medium heat. Add the zucchini, and toss to coat with oil. Cook until just heated through, about 2 to 3 minutes.

4. Transfer to a serving bowl, and pour the sauce over the top and toss before serving.

ROASTED VEGETABLE LETTUCE WRAPS

If you are looking for a simple way to use up your leftover vegetables, try roasting them and then rolling them up in a lettuce wrap. A drizzle of homemade cilantro lime coconut cream sauce adds extra flavor.

Makes 4 (1-wrap) servings

FOR THE SAUCE

½ cup canned coconut milk

¼ cup chopped fresh cilantro

1–2 tablespoons fresh lime juice

1–2 teaspoons agave

pinch of iodized salt

FOR THE LETTUCE WRAPS

1 small zucchini, halved width-wise and sliced into ¼-inch rounds

8 spears asparagus, ends trimmed and quartered

1 small yellow onion, thickly sliced

2 portobello mushroom caps, stems removed, halved and thickly sliced

1 medium beet, peeled, halved, and thinly sliced

2 tablespoons extra virgin olive oil

1 tablespoon red wine vinegar

1 teaspoon dried oregano

6 large leaves green leaf lettuce, stems trimmed

iodized salt and pepper

1. Preheat the oven to 450°F, and line a rimmed baking sheet with foil.

2. To make the sauce, whisk together the coconut milk, cilantro, lime juice, and agave in a medium bowl. Season with a pinch of salt, then set aside.

3. To make the roasted vegetables for the wraps, combine the zucchini, asparagus, onion, mushrooms, and beets in a large bowl. Toss with the olive oil, red wine vinegar, and oregano. Season with salt and pepper to taste.

4. Spread the vegetables in a single layer on the baking sheet. Roast for 10 to 12 minutes, then flip the vegetables with a spatula. Let roast for another 10 to 15 minutes, until tender. Remove from the oven, and cool slightly.

5. To assemble, lay the lettuce leaves flat, and add about one-quarter of the roasted vegetable mixture down the middle. Drizzle with sauce to serve.

GRILLED ROSEMARY VEGETABLE KEBABS

Skewered on fresh rosemary stems, these grilled vegetable kebabs are one of my favorite summer recipes. Feel free to use your favorite vegetables or whatever vegetables you happen to have on hand—it's hard to go wrong with grilled vegetables with that hint of rosemary.

Makes 4 (2-skewer) servings

¼ cup plus 2 tablespoons extra virgin olive oil

1 tablespoon red wine vinegar

1 teaspoon raw honey or agave

8 large sprigs fresh rosemary

1 medium zucchini, cut into 1-inch chunks

1–2 cups whole white mushrooms

1 large yellow onion, cut into 1-inch chunks

iodized salt and pepper

1. To make the marinade, whisk together the olive oil, red wine vinegar, honey or agave, and salt and pepper to taste in a large bowl.

2. Pluck the leaves from the rosemary sprigs, and reserve the stems to use as skewers. Chop the leaves, and add them to the marinade. Toss the zucchini, mushrooms, and onion with the marinade, then cover the bowl. Let the vegetables marinate at room temperature while soaking the rosemary skewers in water for about an hour.

3. Preheat the grill to high heat, and brush the grates with olive oil. If preparing on the stovetop, grease a grill pan with olive oil cooking spray and preheat over high heat.

4. Slide the vegetable chunks onto the soaked rosemary skewers, and shake off the excess marinade. Place on the grill, and cook for 8 to 10 minutes, turning every 2 to 3 minutes, until the vegetables are tender. Transfer the skewers to a serving dish, and drizzle with the remaining marinade. Serve hot.

CHAPTER 10
Side Dishes

BALSAMIC ROASTED BEETS

Fresh beets are a natural source of betaine, a special nutrient that helps to reduce inflammation and protect internal organs, making beets a powerful ally for people with autoimmune disease. Make this recipe vegan-friendly by swapping the honey for pure maple syrup or agave. This side dish pairs well with roasted meat dishes like Garlic Herb Roasted Pork Tenderloin (page 128).

Makes 6 (½-cup) servings

8 medium beets

3 tablespoons extra virgin olive oil

½ teaspoon iodized salt

¼ teaspoon freshly ground pepper

½ cup balsamic vinegar

1½ tablespoons raw honey

1 teaspoon freshly grated orange zest

1. Preheat the oven to 425°F, and line a rimmed baking sheet with foil.

2. Scrub the beets well, and trim the ends. Cut in half and then into ¼-inch-thick slices.

3. Toss with the olive oil, salt, and pepper in a large bowl, and spread on the baking sheet. Roast for 30 to 45 minutes, until just tender, then remove from the oven.

4. Make the glaze by whisking together the balsamic vinegar, honey, and orange zest in a small saucepan over medium-high heat. Bring to a slow boil, then simmer for 5 to 10 minutes, until thick and syrupy.

5. Transfer the beets to a serving bowl, and drizzle with balsamic glaze to serve.

CRANBERRY APRICOT CHUTNEY

For a simple side dish, on the edge of sweet and tart, try this cranberry apricot chutney. Serve it with your favorite roasted meat or Coconut Mixed Vegetable Curry (page 153). Rich in iodine, cranberries are also among the best sources of antioxidants and natural anti-inflammatory compounds. Apricots are also rich in antioxidants and are particularly high in vitamin C, vitamin A, potassium, and copper.

Makes 8 to 10 (¼-cup) servings

2 tablespoons coconut oil

½ small sweet onion, diced

1 clove garlic, minced

¾ teaspoon ground cinnamon

¼ teaspoon ground cloves

1 pound fresh or frozen cranberries, rinsed well

1 cup chopped dried apricots

½ cup pure maple syrup

¼ cup apple cider vinegar

¼ cup water

1 tablespoon fresh lemon juice

iodized salt and pepper

1. Heat the coconut oil in a medium saucepan over medium-high heat. Add the onion and garlic, and cook until softened, about 3 minutes, stirring often. Stir in the cinnamon and cloves, and cook for 2 minutes more. Add the cranberries, apricots, maple syrup, and apple cider vinegar. Stir in the water, and simmer for 5 minutes, or until the cranberries start to burst.

2. Gently mash some of the cranberries with the back of a wooden spoon, and continue to cook until thickened, about 5 minutes more. Stir in the lemon juice, and season with salt and pepper to taste. Serve warm.

CILANTRO LIME CUCUMBER RED ONION SALAD

For a simple salad full of fresh flavor, look no further than this recipe. Cilantro is what gives the salad its fresh flavor, and it also adds some key nutrients including antioxidants, vitamins A and K, and several essential minerals. For a complete meal, serve the salad with Ginger Grilled Zucchini Steaks (page 145) or Balsamic Grilled Portobello Caps (page 151).

Makes 4 (1-cup) servings

¼ cup fresh lime juice (from about 2 large limes)

2 tablespoons extra virgin olive oil

1 clove garlic, minced

2 medium seedless cucumbers, thinly sliced

1 small red onion, thinly sliced

¼ cup chopped fresh cilantro

iodized salt and pepper

1. In a large bowl, whisk together the lime juice, olive oil, garlic, and salt and pepper to taste. Add the sliced cucumber, red onion, and fresh cilantro, and toss to coat.

2. Cover and chill the salad in the refrigerator for 30 minutes before serving.

HONEY DILL BABY CARROTS

These carrots are sweet and tender with just the right amount of bite, and they pair well with roasted meats like Garlic Herb Roasted Pork Tenderloin (page 128). Carrots contain a number of powerful antioxidants including carotenoids such as beta-carotene and lutein. The high antioxidant content means that carrots can help to improve cardiovascular health while also helping to reduce the risk for certain types of cancer.

Makes 6 to 8 (½-cup) servings

1½ pounds fresh baby carrots

1½ tablespoons coconut oil

2 tablespoons raw honey

2 tablespoons chopped fresh dill

iodized salt and pepper

1. Fill a medium saucepan with 1½ inches of water, and place a metal steamer insert inside. Bring the water to a boil over high heat, then add the carrots to the steamer basket. Cover the saucepan, and steam the carrots for 15 to 20 minutes, until tender. Transfer to a serving dish.

2. Melt the coconut oil in a medium skillet over medium heat. Add the honey and dill, and cook until the honey is melted, about 2 minutes, stirring often. Add the steamed carrots to the skillet, season with salt and pepper to taste, then toss to coat and serve hot.

LACTO-FERMENTED FRUIT AND VEGETABLE MEDLEY

In addition to increasing the shelf life of the fruit and vegetables, the process of fermentation actually improves the nutrient content of the ingredients by increasing the amount of beneficial enzymes and vitamin B. Serve these vegetables as a side with your favorite sandwich or enjoy them as a snack.

Makes about 16 (½-cup) servings

2 cups sweet red apples, diced

2 cups carrots, peeled and thinly sliced

3–4 medium beets, peeled and diced

3–4 medium parsnips, peeled and thinly sliced

2–3 tablespoons grated fresh ginger

1 tablespoon coarse sea salt plus more as needed

up to 4 cups warm filtered water as needed

1. Combine the apples, carrots, beets, parsnips, and ginger in a large bowl. Sprinkle with 1 tablespoon of sea salt, and toss the ingredients together.

2. Pack into a half-gallon glass jar, pounding with a wooden spoon to release the liquid in the vegetables.

3. If the natural juices don't fill the jar within 1 inch of the top, combine 2 tablespoons of sea salt with 4 cups of warm filtered water, and use as much as needed to fill the jar.

4. Place the lid tightly on the jar and set in a cool area for 3 to 5 days, until fermented.

5. Taste-test the vegetables after 3 days. If they are not tart enough to your liking, allow to ferment longer. Once the vegetables have reached the desired level of sourness, transfer to the refrigerator. The fermented vegetables will keep for 3 to 6 months.

LACTO-FERMENTED CARROTS

The process of lacto-fermentation gives these carrot sticks a kick of tangy flavor and a boost of nutrition as well because fermented foods contain beneficial bacteria which act as natural probiotics, helping to heal the gut and restore healthy digestion. Serve them as a cold side dish with Coconut Flour Balsamic Veggie Wraps (page 107) or simply enjoy them as a healthy snack.

Makes 8 (½-cup) servings

2–3 tablespoons coarse sea salt

2 cups filtered water

4 cloves garlic

1½ pounds baby carrots

1. To make the brine, in a large bowl whisk together the sea salt and water until fully dissolved.

2. Place the garlic cloves in the bottom of a quart glass jar.

3. Pack the carrots vertically into the jar so they reach to about 1½ inches below the mouth.

4. Pour in enough brine to completely cover the carrots, leaving about 1 inch of space at the top. Cover the jar tightly with the lid, and place in a cool location to rest for 7 to 10 days.

5. Taste-test the carrots after 7 days. Let them ferment longer if needed, to reach the desired level of acidity.

6. Once the carrots have finished fermenting, place the jar in the refrigerator. The carrots will keep for 3 to 6 months.

OVEN-ROASTED ACORN SQUASH

This oven-roasted acorn squash is lightly sweetened with maple syrup and roasted until tender—it pairs well with poultry dishes like Whole Roasted Lemon Garlic Chicken (page 122). Fresh acorn squash is an excellent source of gluten-free, grain-free carbohydrate and dietary fiber—it is also rich in vitamin C, zinc, magnesium, and a number of antioxidants.

Makes 4 servings

2 medium acorn squash

2 tablespoons extra virgin olive oil

1–2 tablespoons pure maple syrup

iodized salt and pepper

1. Preheat the oven to 375°F, and line a rimmed baking sheet with foil.

2. Cut the squash in half from stem to tip, then scoop out and discard the seeds.

3. Whisk together the olive oil and maple syrup, and brush the mixture on the cut sides. Season lightly with salt and pepper to taste. Place cut side down on the baking sheet. Roast for 45 to 55 minutes, until tender and caramelized around the edges.

4. Serve in the squash halves, or scoop the flesh into a bowl and mash before serving.

GARLIC GRILLED ASPARAGUS

This tasty summer dish goes well with just about any entree, though the crispness of the asparagus pairs particularly well with tender grilled fish like Grilled Salmon Fillets with Basil Artichoke Pesto (page 111). Asparagus is packed with dietary fiber, vitamins A and C, and antioxidants. It also contains folate, a vitamin known to help boost cognitive performance.

Makes 6 servings

¼ cup extra virgin olive oil

1 tablespoon minced fresh garlic

2 pounds fresh asparagus, ends trimmed

iodized salt and pepper

1. Preheat a grill to high heat, and brush the grates with olive oil. If preparing on the stovetop, grease a grill pan with olive oil cooking spray and preheat over high heat.

2. Combine the olive oil and garlic in a shallow dish. Add the trimmed asparagus, turning to coat, then season with salt and pepper to taste. Let sit at room temperature for about 15 minutes.

3. Place the asparagus spears on the grill perpendicular to the grates. Grill for 4 to 8 minutes, turning every 2 to 3 minutes, until just tender.

HOMEMADE DILL PICKLES

These homemade pickles are a natural probiotic and their crisp, tangy flavor will rival even the best store-bought pickles! Cucumbers have a very high water content, making them a powerful detoxifier, and they are rich in dietary fiber, magnesium, potassium, and essential vitamins. The grape leaves in this recipe are available at specialty food stores.

Makes about 16 to 20 (1-pickle) servings

5 tablespoons coarse sea salt

8 cups filtered water

5 grape leaves, torn in half

8 cloves garlic

2 large sprigs fresh dill, coarsely chopped

1–2 teaspoons whole black peppercorns

4 pounds pickling cucumbers

1. To make the brine, in a large bowl whisk together the sea salt and water until dissolved. Set aside.

2. Place half of the grape leaves, garlic, dill, and peppercorns in a half-gallon glass jar.

3. Trim the ends from the pickling cucumbers, and pack half of them tightly into the jar.

4. Add the remaining grape leaves, garlic, dill, and peppercorns, then pack in the rest of the cucumbers.

5. Pour in the brine, leaving about 1 to 2 inches of space at the top of the jar. Cover the jar tightly with the lid, and set in a cool place for at least 48 hours.

6. Taste-test the pickles after 48 hours. If not acidic enough, allow to pickle longer. Once the desired level of acidity is reached, transfer to the refrigerator. Pickles will keep for 3 to 6 months in the refrigerator.

BLANCHED GREEN BEANS WITH BACON DRESSING

These green beans are tossed with a warm bacon dressing and mixed with chopped bacon bits, making for an indulgent side dish you won't be able to get enough of. These crisp vegetables are rich in dietary fiber and protein. They also contain a significant amount of vitamin C, magnesium, calcium, and B vitamins.

Makes 6 to 8 (½-cup) servings

2 pounds fresh green beans, ends trimmed

6–8 slices uncured bacon

1 small yellow onion, diced

2 cloves garlic, minced

2½ tablespoons apple cider vinegar

2 tablespoons extra virgin olive oil

iodized salt and pepper

1. Bring a large pot of salted water to a boil over high heat. Add the green beans, and cook for 4 to 5 minutes, until just tender. Drain the beans, and immediately run cold water over them to stop the cooking. Transfer to a medium bowl.

2. Heat the bacon in a large skillet over medium-high heat, and cook until crisp, about 4 to 5 minutes. Transfer to paper towels to drain, then chop coarsely.

3. Reserve 2 tablespoons of bacon grease from the skillet, and keep the rest for use in other recipes. Reheat the reserved grease over medium heat. Add the onion and garlic, and cook for 4 to 6 minutes until the onions are translucent. Stir in the apple cider vinegar and olive oil, then season with salt and pepper to taste. Stir in the green beans and cooked bacon, and cook until just heated through. Serve hot.

WINTER ROOT VEGETABLE RAGOUT

Loaded with dietary fiber and essential nutrients, this is a power-packed, hearty side dish. Feel free to substitute any vegetables from the approved vegetables food list (page 54) if you prefer.

Makes 8 (1-cup) servings

2 medium yellow onions, chopped

2 pounds turnips, peeled and chopped

2 large parsnips, peeled and chopped

½ pound chopped carrots

1 medium celery root, peeled and chopped

2 medium leeks, chopped (white and light green parts only)

2 tablespoons extra virgin olive oil

2 teaspoons chopped fresh rosemary

1 teaspoon chopped fresh thyme

1½ cups vegetable broth

iodized salt and pepper

1. Preheat the oven to 475°F, and line a rimmed baking sheet with foil.

2. Combine the onions, turnips, parsnips, carrots, celery root, and leeks in a large bowl. Toss with the olive oil, rosemary, and thyme. Season with salt and pepper to taste. Spread the vegetables on the baking sheet, and roast for 25 to 30 minutes, turning every 10 minutes, until tender and browned.

3. Bring the vegetable broth to a simmer in a large saucepan over medium-high heat. Add the cooked vegetables, and simmer for 5 to 10 minutes, until tender. Adjust the seasoning to taste, and serve hot.

GARLIC SAUTÉED SPINACH

If you are looking for a tasty side dish that is quick and easy to prepare, consider this garlic sautéed spinach. Tossed with coconut oil and slices of fresh garlic, this sautéed spinach is tender and flavorful—it pairs perfectly with roasted meats like Maple Lime Chicken Drumsticks (page 126).

Makes about 6 (1-cup) servings

2 tablespoons coconut oil

3 cloves garlic, thinly sliced

2½ pounds fresh spinach, coarsely chopped

iodized salt and pepper

1. Heat the coconut oil in a large skillet over medium heat.

2. Add the garlic, and cook for 2 to 3 minutes, until it starts to brown. Use a slotted spoon to transfer the garlic to a paper towel to drain.

3. Add the spinach to the hot skillet then cover and cook for 3 to 5 minutes, until the spinach is just wilted. Season with salt and pepper to taste, and transfer to a serving bowl. Sprinkle the cooked garlic over the top to serve.

GOITROGEN ALERT:
max 6 to 8 servings
per week

LEMON GARLIC SPAGHETTI SQUASH

If you find yourself missing pasta on the Hashimoto's diet, this lemon garlic spaghetti squash is a side dish you'll definitely want to try. Full of fresh garlic flavor and shredded into threads that resemble angel hair pasta, this spaghetti squash dish is a perfect pasta alternative.

Makes 6 to 8 (½-cup) servings

1 large (6 to 8 pound) spaghetti squash

extra virgin olive oil, as needed

¼ cup coconut oil

1 small yellow onion, diced

1 tablespoon minced fresh garlic

¼ cup fresh lemon juice

1 tablespoon fresh lemon zest

iodized salt and pepper

1. Preheat the oven to 400°F, and line a rimmed baking sheet with foil.

2. Cut the spaghetti squash in half lengthwise then scoop out and discard the seeds. Brush the cut sides with olive oil, and season with salt and pepper to taste. Place the halves cut side down on the baking sheet. Roast for about 20 minutes, until the squash can be pierced easily with a knife.

3. Remove from the oven, and let sit until cool enough to handle. Shred the flesh with a fork, scoop into a large bowl, and set aside.

4. Melt the coconut oil in a large skillet over medium-high heat. Add the onion and garlic, and cook for 5 to 6 minutes, until tender. Stir in the cooked spaghetti squash, lemon juice, and lemon zest, and cook until heated through. Season with salt and pepper to taste. Serve hot.

TROPICAL JICAMA SALAD WITH LIME VINAIGRETTE

Jicama is a crisp, sweet vegetable—with a unique flavor and texture—that many people overlook. It is also rich in dietary fiber as well as a number of essential minerals including iron, magnesium, and copper.

Serves 6 to 8 (½-cup) servings

1 large jicama, peeled and diced

1 large ripe mango, diced

2 ripe kiwi, peeled and sliced

½ small red onion, diced

¼ cup fresh lime juice (from about 2 large limes)

¼ cup raw honey

1 tablespoon extra virgin olive oil

½ cup chopped fresh cilantro

iodized salt and pepper

1. Combine the jicama, mango, kiwi, and red onion in a medium bowl.

2. Make the vinaigrette by whisking together the lime juice, honey, and olive oil in a small bowl. Toss the jicama mixture with the vinaigrette and the cilantro. Season with salt and pepper to taste.

3. Cover the bowl with plastic wrap, and chill in the refrigerator for at least 15 minutes before serving.

MANGO PINEAPPLE SALSA WITH CILANTRO

This salsa is a fresh and fruity side dish that goes particularly well with baked fish and chicken. Loaded with tropical fruit flavor and fresh cilantro, the dish is tasty and easy to prepare. You can make it up to 24 hours ahead so the flavors have plenty of time to combine.

Makes 8 to 10 (¼-cup) servings

1½ cups chopped fresh mango

1 cup chopped fresh pineapple

1 medium ripe peach, chopped

½ cup diced jicama

¼–½ cup chopped fresh cilantro

2 green onions, white and green parts only, thinly sliced

2 tablespoons fresh lime juice

1 teaspoon raw honey (optional)

1. Combine the mango, pineapple, peach, and jicama in a large bowl. Add the cilantro, green onions, lime juice, and honey, if using, and toss to combine. Cover the bowl with plastic wrap, and chill in the refrigerator for at least 1 hour so the flavors can meld.

2. Serve chilled or at room temperature.

CHAPTER 11
Snacks

TROPICAL FRUIT SALAD WITH LEMON COCONUT CREAM

This tropical fruit salad pairs perfectly with fresh lemon coconut cream and toasted coconut flakes. You can customize this recipe with your favorite or seasonal fruits. If you like your coconut cream a little sweeter, add a teaspoon or two of raw honey.

Makes 6 to 8 servings (serving size is ½ cup fruit salad plus 2 tablespoons coconut cream)

FOR THE FRUIT SALAD

2 tablespoons raw honey

2 tablespoons fresh lime juice

1 tablespoon fresh lime zest

2 tablespoons chopped fresh mint leaves

1 ripe mango, chopped

½ fresh pineapple, cored and chopped

2 ripe kiwi, peeled and sliced

1 large ripe banana, sliced

1 cup unsweetened shredded coconut

FOR THE COCONUT CREAM

2 (14-ounce) cans coconut milk, refrigerated overnight

2–3 tablespoons fresh lemon juice

1. Preheat the oven to 350°F.

2. To make the fruit salad dressing, whisk together the honey, lime juice, lime zest, and mint in a large bowl. Add the mango,

pineapple, kiwi, and banana. Toss well to coat. Set aside to allow the fruits to absorb the dressing.

3. Spread the shredded coconut on a rimmed baking sheet, and toast in the oven for 5 minutes, until golden brown. Remove from the oven, and set aside to cool.

4. To make the coconut cream, open the cans of coconut milk from the bottom and spoon the solids into a large bowl. Discard the liquid or save it for another recipe. Add the lemon juice, and beat with a whisk or an electric mixer until thick and creamy, about 2 minutes.

5. To serve, top the fruit salad with a dollop of coconut cream, and garnish with toasted coconut flakes.

BANANA CINNAMON
PROTEIN SHAKE

This vegan-friendly protein shake is thick and creamy, and loaded with fresh banana flavor and a hint of cinnamon. Feel free to sweeten this shake with a little pure maple syrup.

Makes 2 (8- to 12-ounce) servings

2 small frozen bananas, sliced

1 cup canned coconut milk

1½ cups coconut water

½ cup ice cubes

1 scoop vanilla vegan protein powder

½ teaspoon ground cinnamon, plus extra to sprinkle on top

2 slices fresh banana, to garnish

1. Combine the frozen bananas, coconut milk, and coconut water in a blender. Pulse several times to chop. Add the ice cubes, protein powder, and cinnamon. Blend on high speed for 30 to 60 seconds, until smooth.

2. Pour into two large glasses. Sprinkle with a little extra cinnamon, and garnish with a slice of fresh banana.

CUCUMBER MELON PROTEIN SHAKE

Both fresh cucumber and honeydew melon are powerful detoxifiers that can help to cleanse your digestive system in preparation for the gut-healing benefits of the Hashimoto's diet.

Makes 2 (8- to 12-ounce) servings

½ cup chopped seedless cucumber, plus extra to garnish

½ cup chopped fresh honeydew, plus extra to garnish

½ small frozen banana, sliced

1 cup coconut water

1 cup ice cubes

1 scoop vanilla vegan protein powder

¼ cup chopped fresh mint leaves

1. Place the cucumber, honeydew, banana, and coconut water in a blender. Pulse several times to chop. Add the ice cubes, protein powder, and mint. Blend on high speed for 30 to 60 seconds, until smooth and well combined.

2. Pour into two large glasses. Cut halfway into two cucumber slices and melon wedges and place them on the rim of each glass to garnish.

TROPICAL MANGO LIME PROTEIN SHAKE

Made with tropical fruits and creamy coconut milk, this shake is packed with flavor and nutrients. Fresh kiwi is a natural source of potassium, manganese, and dietary fiber, while mango is rich in antioxidants and immune-boosting vitamin C. Banana, in addition to contributing to the smooth texture of this protein shake, adds its own boost of potassium as well as copper and biotin.

Makes 2 (8- to 12-ounce) servings

1 ripe kiwi, peeled and sliced

1 cup frozen chopped mango

½ small frozen banana, sliced

1 cup canned coconut milk

½ cup ice cubes

2–3 tablespoons fresh lime juice

1 scoop vanilla vegan protein powder

¼ teaspoon coconut extract

2 lime wedges to garnish

1. Place the kiwi, mango, banana, and coconut milk in a blender. Pulse several times to chop. Add the ice cubes, lime juice, protein powder, and coconut extract. Blend on high speed for 30 to 60 seconds, until smooth and well combined.

2. Pour into two large glasses, and garnish with a lime wedge.

GINGER PEAR PROTEIN SMOOTHIE

Ginger is a powerful superfood (a food that is particularly high in various nutrients), loaded with spicy flavor and health benefits. In addition to being a natural anti-inflammatory, ginger can help to stabilize blood sugar and blood cholesterol levels.

Makes 2 (8- to 12-ounce) servings

1 small frozen banana, sliced

½ cup sliced fresh pear, plus extra to garnish

1 cup unsweetened apple juice

1 cup ice cubes

1 scoop vanilla vegan protein powder

½ teaspoon grated fresh ginger

¼ teaspoon ground cinnamon, plus extra for sprinkling on top

1. Combine the frozen banana, pear, and apple juice in a blender. Pulse several times to chop. Add the ice, protein powder, ginger, and cinnamon. Blend on high speed for 30 to 60 seconds, until smooth.

2. Pour into two large glasses. Sprinkle with ground cinnamon, and garnish the rim of each glass with a slice of fresh pear.

GOITROGEN ALERT:
max 6 to 8 servings
per week

AVOCADO HONEYDEW SMOOTHIE

Sweet, thick, and creamy, this smoothie is rich in monounsaturated fats from avocado as well as potassium, vitamin C, and B vitamins from the melon. Enjoy this smoothie fresh for the best health benefits.

Makes 2 (8- to 12-ounce) servings

1 cup chopped fresh honeydew

½ small avocado

1 cup unsweetened apple juice or water

½ cup Homemade Coconut Yogurt (page 66)

½ cup ice cubes

1 tablespoon agave or raw honey

1 teaspoon fresh lime juice

1. Place all of the ingredients in a blender. Blend until smooth and well combined.

2. Pour into two large glasses.

BLUEBERRY SUPERFOOD SMOOTHIE

Although this smoothie is made with beet greens and spirulina, all you will taste is the sweetness of the blueberries and banana. This recipe includes a variety of superfoods—that is, foods particularly high in essential nutrients. In addition to antioxidant-rich blueberries, the smoothie contains protein-packed beet greens and shredded coconut, plus iodine-rich spirulina powder.

Makes 2 (8- to 12-ounce) servings

1 cup frozen blueberries

1 small frozen banana, sliced

1 cup chopped fresh beet greens

1 cup unsweetened apple juice or coconut water

½ cup canned coconut milk

½ cup ice cubes

¼ cup unsweetened shredded coconut

1 teaspoon dried spirulina powder

1. Combine the blueberries, banana, beet greens, and apple juice in a blender, and blend at high speed until smooth. Add the remaining ingredients, and pulse several times to chop. Then blend for 30 to 60 seconds on high speed, until smooth and well combined.

2. Pour into two glasses.

GREEN TEA PROTEIN SMOOTHIE

Matcha is a finely ground powder made from a special type of green tea available at specialty food stores and tea shops. It's loaded with antioxidants and also has a high theanine content, which helps to improve mental focus. The caffeine and theanine in matcha powder combine to give you a boost of energy without the crash you might get from other caffeinated drinks like coffee.

Makes 2 (8- to 12-ounce) servings

1 small frozen banana, sliced

½ large ripe avocado, chopped

1 cup canned coconut milk

½ cup ice cubes

1 scoop vanilla vegan protein powder

1 teaspoon matcha green tea powder

2 slices fresh banana, to garnish

1. Place the banana, avocado, and coconut milk in a blender. Pulse several times to chop. Add the ice cubes, protein powder, and green tea powder. Blend on high speed for 30 to 60 seconds, until smooth and well combined.

2. Pour into two large glasses, and garnish the rim of each glass with a slice of banana.

CRAN-GRAPE MORNING SMOOTHIE

Using frozen green grapes instead of ice cubes gives this cran-grape morning smoothie plenty of natural sweetness. This nutritious vegan smoothie is also loaded with antioxidants, vitamin C, and manganese, as well as dietary fiber. It's the perfect way to start your day.

Makes 2 (8- to 12-ounce) servings

1 cup frozen green grapes

½ cup frozen cranberries

1 small frozen banana, sliced

1 cup unsweetened cranberry or grape juice

½ cup Homemade Coconut Yogurt (page 66)

1 teaspoon agave

⅛ teaspoon ground cinnamon or ground ginger

1. Place all of the ingredients in a blender, and pulse several times to chop. Blend on high speed for 30 to 60 seconds, until smooth and well combined.

2. Pour into two glasses.

STRAWBERRY KIWI SMOOTHIE

If you find yourself in need of a nutrient-rich snack that will also help you meet your daily fiber recommendations, consider this strawberry kiwi smoothie. If you use fresh strawberries instead of frozen, add an extra half cup of ice.

Makes 2 (8- to 12-ounce) servings

1 cup frozen sliced strawberries

2 ripe kiwi, peeled and sliced

1 handful fresh spinach

1 cup canned coconut milk

½ cup ice cubes

1 tablespoon coconut oil

1 teaspoon raw honey

1. Place the strawberries, kiwi, spinach, and coconut milk in a blender. Pulse several times to chop. Add the ice cubes, coconut oil, and honey. Blend on high speed for 30 to 60 seconds, until smooth and well combined.

2. Pour into two large glasses.

GOITROGEN ALERT:
max 6 to 8 servings
per week

AVOCADO COCONUT PROTEIN SMOOTHIE

Thick and creamy, this smoothie offers a powerful combination of healthy fats. This smoothie also contains spirulina powder, which is rich in iron, magnesium, and a number of B vitamins.

Makes 2 (8- to 12-ounce) servings

½ large ripe avocado, chopped

1 small frozen banana, sliced

1 cup canned coconut milk

½ cup ice cubes

1 scoop vanilla vegan protein powder

¼ cup unsweetened shredded coconut, plus more for sprinkling

½ teaspoon dried spirulina powder

1. Place the avocado, banana, and coconut milk in a blender. Pulse several times to chop. Add the ice cubes, protein powder, shredded coconut, and spirulina powder. Blend on high speed for 30 to 60 seconds, until smooth and well combined.

2. Pour into two large glasses, and sprinkle with unsweetened shredded coconut.

BAKED BUTTERNUT SQUASH FRIES

Flavored with oregano and tossed with olive oil, these baked butternut squash fries are just as satisfying as traditional potato fries, but they are much healthier! Butternut squash is a gluten-free, grain-free carbohydrate rich in dietary fiber, beta-carotene, folate, and antioxidant compounds. Cut into wedges and baked in a hot oven, it makes fries that are crisp on the outside and tender in the middle.

Makes 4 (½-cup) servings

1 large butternut squash

3–4 tablespoons extra virgin olive oil

2 teaspoons dried oregano

1 teaspoon iodized salt

½ teaspoon freshly ground black pepper

1. Preheat the oven to 425°F, and line a baking sheet with parchment paper.

2. Cut the squash in half, then scoop out and discard the seeds. Use a sharp knife to cut away the peel. Cut the flesh into wedges no more than ½ inch thick. Place the squash wedges in a large bowl, and toss with the olive oil, oregano, salt, and pepper.

3. Spread the wedges in a single layer on the baking sheet. Bake for 22 to 25 minutes, until crisp and golden brown. Cool slightly before serving.

SALTED GARLIC NORI CHIPS

Nori is a type of seaweed traditionally used for sushi, but it can also be used to make crunchy, salty baked chips which can be served with homemade salsa or Avocado Zucchini Hummus (page 191). Along with being an excellent source of iodine, nori is loaded with vitamin B12, dietary fiber, and vegetarian protein.

Makes 4 to 6 (8- to 10-chip) servings

12 sheets nori

water, as needed

1 tablespoon extra virgin olive oil

2 cloves garlic, minced

iodized salt

1. Preheat the oven to 275°F, and line two baking sheets with parchment paper.

2. Lay six sheets of nori on a flat surface. Lightly brush with water, then place a second sheet on top of each. Press the sheets together gently by hand. Use a sharp knife to cut the layered sheets horizontally into ½-inch strips, then cut each strip in half.

3. Arrange the strips of nori on the baking sheets so the edges do not touch. Place in a single layer with the shiny side up.

4. Whisk together the olive oil and garlic in a small bowl. Brush the strips, then sprinkle lightly with salt, as desired, keeping in mind that nori itself is salty.

5. Bake for 15 to 20 minutes, until crisp and dark green. Remove from the oven, and let cool on the baking sheets. Store the extras in an airtight container for up to 7 days.

GARLIC BAKED ZUCCHINI CHIPS

These baked zucchini chips are thinly sliced, perfectly crisp, and absolutely irresistible. The zucchini is a good source of magnesium and potassium, and the fresh garlic—which adds lots of flavor—is an antioxidant, anti-inflammatory, and immune booster. Serve these chips on their own or pair them with some Avocado Zucchini Hummus (page 191) for dipping!

Makes 3 to 4 (½-cup) servings

2 medium zucchini

1–2 tablespoons extra virgin olive oil

garlic powder

iodized salt and pepper

1. Preheat the oven to 225°F, and line a baking sheet with parchment paper.

2. Slice the zucchini as thinly as possible, using a mandolin if you have one. Lay the zucchini slices on paper towels, and sprinkle lightly with salt. Let rest for 10 minutes, then blot dry.

3. Arrange in a single layer on the baking sheet. Brush lightly with olive oil, then season to taste with garlic powder, salt, and pepper. Bake for about 2 hours, until crisp and dried. Let cool on the baking sheet before serving. Store the extras in an airtight container for up to 7 days.

CANDIED SWEET POTATO SLICES

This is a sweet, indulgent snack that happens to be loaded with manganese, potassium, and B vitamins.

Makes 10 to 12 (2- to 3-slice) servings

1 pound sweet potatoes, peeled and ends trimmed

¼ cup coconut oil

¾ cup raw honey or pure maple syrup

1. Place the sweet potatoes in a large saucepan, and cover with water. Bring to a boil over medium-high heat, and simmer until cooked halfway.

2. Pour off the water from the saucepan, and run cold water over the sweet potatoes until cool. Drain, cut into ½-inch slices, and set aside.

3. Melt the coconut oil in a large, deep skillet over medium-high heat, then whisk in the honey or maple syrup. Reduce the heat and simmer the mixture on low heat until it thickens into a glaze. Add the sweet potato slices in a single layer, and simmer until the edges darken. Flip the slices, and simmer until cooked through. Transfer to a wire rack set over a baking sheet, and allow the excess glaze to drip off.

4. Let cool, then enjoy a few slices as an occasional treat. Store the extras in an airtight container for up to 7 days.

GOITROGEN ALERT:
max 6 to 8 servings
per week

AVOCADO ZUCCHINI HUMMUS

Traditionally, hummus is made with chickpeas and sesame tahini, neither of which is included in the Hashimoto's diet. This recipe is not only completely vegan, Paleo, and gluten-free, but it tastes just like regular hummus. Serve it with Garlic Baked Zucchini Chips (page 189) for dipping!

Makes 8 to 10 (¼-cup) servings

10 to 12 ounces fresh zucchini, peeled and chopped

1 medium ripe avocado, chopped

3 cloves garlic, chopped

¼ cup coconut oil or 2 tablespoons extra virgin olive oil

2 tablespoons fresh lemon juice

iodized salt

ground white pepper

1. Place the zucchini, avocado, and garlic in a food processor. Pulse several times until finely chopped. Add the oil, lemon juice, salt, and pepper to taste. Blend until the mixture is smooth and creamy, adding a little water, if needed, to thin.

2. Spoon the hummus into a bowl, and serve with fresh sliced vegetables or Garlic Baked Zucchini Chips.

PROSCIUTTO WRAPPED ASPARAGUS SPEARS

Fresh prosciutto is somewhat of a delicacy, and it's chewy, crunchy texture pairs nicely with tender, blanched asparagus. Asparagus is rich in dietary fiber, folate and other vitamins, and chromium, a trace mineral that helps to regulate the metabolism. In addition to being rich in protein, prosciutto also contains trace amounts of iron, zinc, and vitamin B12.

Makes 8 to 10 (3- to 4-spear) servings

1½ pounds fresh asparagus

1 tablespoon melted coconut oil

6–8 ounces grass-fed thinly sliced prosciutto, halved lengthwise

iodized salt and pepper

1. Preheat the broiler to the highest heat setting, and place an oven rack about 6 inches below the element. Line a baking sheet with parchment paper.

2. Trim the ends of the asparagus, and arrange the spears in a single layer on the baking sheet. Drizzle the coconut oil over the spears, and season with salt and pepper to taste. Gently toss by hand until evenly coated, then transfer to a large plate.

3. One at a time, wrap the pieces of prosciutto around the asparagus spears, starting just under the tip. Place the prosciutto-wrapped spears on the baking sheet as you finish them, leaving just a little space between them.

4. Broil for about 3 minutes, then flip the spears and broil for another 2 to 3 minutes, until crisp and browned. Remove from the oven, and allow to cool slightly before serving.

FRIED SQUASH FRITTERS WITH DILL SAUCE

These squash fritters have a crispy, crunchy exterior and a tender center. Serve them with a dollop of creamy dill sauce, and you have the ideal snack. Feel free to substitute zucchini or add shredded carrot for color to contrast with the yellow or green color of the squash.

Makes 4 servings (serving size is 2 or 3 fritters plus 2 tablespoons sauce)

FOR THE FRITTERS

2 cups finely shredded yellow summer squash

¼ cup sifted coconut flour

2 teaspoons baking powder

½ teaspoon iodized salt

2–3 tablespoons coconut oil

FOR THE DILL SAUCE

1 cup Homemade Coconut Yogurt (page 66)

2 medium green onions, white and green parts only, thinly sliced

1 tablespoon fresh lemon juice

1–2 teaspoons chopped fresh dill

1. Spread the shredded squash on a clean dish towel, roll it up, and wring out as much moisture as you can. Place the squash in a medium bowl. Add the coconut flour, baking powder, and salt. Stir until thoroughly combined. Let rest for 5 minutes at room temperature.

2. Preheat a large skillet over medium heat, and add the coconut oil. Once the oil is melted and hot, spoon the squash mixture into the skillet in ¼-cup portions. Use a fork to spread the mixture to about ¾ inch thick, and cook for 2 to 3 minutes, until the underside is browned. Carefully flip the fritters, and fry for another 1 or 2 minutes, until the bottom is browned. Transfer to paper towels to drain, and repeat with the remaining batter.

3. While the fritters are cooling, make the sauce by combining the coconut yogurt, green onions, lemon juice, and fresh dill in a small bowl. Stir until smooth and well combined. Serve with the warm fritters.

CINNAMON APPLE FRUIT LEATHER

Enjoy the sweetness of fresh apple and the chewiness of a fruit roll without the artificial ingredients by preparing fruit leather right in your own kitchen. Once you get the hang of this recipe, you can try it with other fruits like pears and peaches.

Makes 4 servings

4 cups fresh sweet apples, peeled and chopped

½ cup water

2 tablespoons raw honey or pure maple syrup

1 tablespoon fresh lemon juice

1–2 teaspoons ground cinnamon

1. Place the chopped apples in a medium saucepan, and add the water. Bring to a simmer over medium heat. Cover the saucepan, and cook for 10 to 12 minutes, until tender. Stir in the honey or maple syrup, lemon juice, and cinnamon. Use a potato masher to mash the cooked apples and combine the ingredients.

2. Transfer to a blender, and blend until smooth.

3. Preheat the oven to 170°F, and line a rimmed baking sheet with parchment paper. Spread the pureed mixture as evenly as possible on the baking sheet. Bake for 2 to 3 hours, until the mixture is tacky but not sticky.

4. Cut into four slices, and roll up in strips of parchment paper or plastic wrap to keep them from sticking together.

CHAPTER 12
Desserts

VANILLA COCONUT MILK ICE CREAM

Nothing says indulgent like a bowl of sweet, velvety ice cream. This homemade ice cream is made with canned coconut milk, which makes it a Paleo and dairy-free alternative to traditional ice cream. Feel free to add your favorite mix-ins, like fresh fruit, raisins, or coconut flakes.

Makes 8 (½-cup) servings

2 (14-ounce) cans coconut milk, chilled overnight

½–¾ cup raw honey

1 vanilla bean

1. Open the cans of coconut milk, and spoon the contents into a large bowl. Whisk until smooth, then whisk in the honey a little at a time. Taste after each addition, and keep adding until the mixture reaches the desired level of sweetness.

2. Use a small, sharp knife to slice the vanilla bean down the middle. Scrape the seeds into the bowl, and whisk thoroughly into the mixture.

3. Spoon into a freezer-safe sealable container, and freeze until solid.

4. To serve, thaw for about 10 minutes, until soft enough to scoop.

PEACH LIME SORBET

The natural sweetness of fresh peaches contrasts nicely with the tartness of fresh lime juice in this homemade sorbet. Rich in a variety of nutrients, peaches have significant antioxidant properties as well as anti-cancer, immune-boosting, and cholesterol-lowing benefits.

Makes 8 (½-cup) servings

6–8 ripe peaches, peeled and sliced

1 (14-ounce) can coconut milk

2 tablespoons fresh lime juice

1 teaspoon fresh lime zest

1 teaspoon vanilla extract

1. Place the peaches in a food processor, and blend until pureed. Add the coconut milk, lime juice, lime zest, and vanilla extract. Blend until thoroughly combined.

2. Spoon into a freezer-safe sealable container. Stir about every hour until the sorbet is frozen.

3. Break the frozen sorbet into pieces, and puree in a food processor until smooth, and serve immediately.

GOITROGEN ALERT:
max 6 to 8 servings
per week

POMEGRANATE GINGER SORBET

What better way to cool down on a hot summer day than with a scoop of this sorbet! In addition to giving this recipe a zesty flavor, ginger and pomegranate juice are loaded with healthy nutrients. Pomegranate juice is rich in antioxidants, while ginger is known for its natural anti-inflammatory properties.

Makes about 8 (½-cup) servings

3 cups unsweetened pomegranate juice, divided

½ cup agave

1 tablespoon grated fresh ginger

1. Whisk together 1 cup of the pomegranate juice with the agave and ginger in a small saucepan. Heat the mixture over medium-high heat until boiling, then stir until the agave dissolves completely. Remove from the heat, and let cool to room temperature.

2. Strain the mixture through a sieve into a large bowl. Whisk in the remaining 2 cups of pomegranate juice, then cover the bowl and chill in the refrigerator for at least 2 hours.

3. Spoon into freezer-safe sealable freezer-safe container, and freeze. Stir about every hour until the sorbet is frozen.

4. Break the frozen sorbet into pieces, and puree in a food processor until smooth, and serve immediately.

CINNAMON COCONUT FROZEN YOGURT

Pungent ground cinnamon is one of the healthiest spices on earth. It is an excellent source of antioxidants and has natural anti-inflammatory properties. In this recipe, it has a warming effect on this chilled dessert.

Makes 6 (½-cup) servings

2 cups Homemade Coconut Yogurt (page 66)

1 (14-ounce) can coconut milk

4–6 tablespoons agave

1 teaspoon vanilla extract

1 cup shredded unsweetened coconut

½–1 teaspoon ground cinnamon

1. Whisk together the coconut yogurt and coconut milk in a large bowl. Add the agave and vanilla extract, and whisk until smooth. Stir in the shredded coconut and ground cinnamon until well combined.

2. Spoon into a freezer-safe sealable container, and freeze until solid.

3. To serve, thaw for about 10 minutes, until soft enough to scoop.

LEMON COCONUT CUPCAKES

These homemade cupcakes combine the tartness of lemon with the rich flavor and natural sweetness of shredded coconut. Topped with sweetened coconut milk frosting, these cupcakes are a healthy dessert option you will find yourself making over and over again!

Makes 12 (1-cupcake) servings

FOR THE CUPCAKES

¼ cup agar-agar flakes

¼ cup warm water

½ cup sifted coconut flour

1 tablespoon fresh lemon zest

½ teaspoon baking powder

¼ teaspoon iodized salt

¼ cup plus 2 tablespoons pure maple syrup

¼ cup plus 2 tablespoons melted coconut oil

¼ cup fresh lemon juice

½ cup unsweetened shredded coconut

FOR THE WHIPPED COCONUT CREAM FROSTING

1 (14-ounce) can coconut milk, chilled overnight

2 tablespoons pure maple syrup

1. Preheat the oven to 350°F, and line a regular muffin pan with paper liners.

2. Whisk together the agar-agar flakes and warm water in a large bowl, and set aside.

3. Combine the coconut flour, lemon zest, baking powder, and salt in a medium bowl. In a separate bowl, whisk together the agar-agar mixture, maple syrup, coconut oil, coconut milk, and lemon juice. Whisk the dry ingredients into the wet, until a smooth batter forms, then fold in the shredded coconut.

4. Spoon the batter into the muffin pan, filling each cup about three-quarters full.

5. Bake for 18 to 22 minutes, until a knife inserted in the center comes out clean.

6. Remove from the oven, and cool in the pan for 5 minutes. Transfer the cupcakes to a wire rack to cool completely before frosting.

7. To make the frosting, open the can of coconut milk from the bottom and scoop the coconut milk solids into a medium bowl. Discard the liquid or save it for another recipe. Beat the coconut milk with a hand mixer on high speed for 3 to 5 minutes, until thick and creamy. Fold in the maple syrup, and frost the cupcakes.

8. Spread the frosting on the cooled cupcakes and enjoy!

STRAWBERRY LEMON CUPCAKES

These cupcakes combine sweet strawberries and tart lemons, but if you feel adventurous, try out some other fruit combinations as well. Feel free to swap out the strawberries for whatever type of fruit you choose for a new flavor combination like raspberry lemon or lemon blueberry.

Makes 12 (1-cupcake) servings

¼ cup agar-agar flakes

¼ cup warm water

½ cup sifted coconut flour

1 teaspoon fresh lemon zest

½ teaspoon baking powder

¼ teaspoon iodized salt

½ cup agave

1 tablespoon fresh lemon juice

1 teaspoon vanilla extract

½ cup diced fresh strawberries

1 recipe Whipped Coconut Cream Frosting (page 199)

1. Preheat the oven to 350°F, and line a regular muffin pan with paper liners.

2. Combine the agar-agar flakes and the warm water in a large bowl, then set aside. Whisk together the coconut flour, lemon zest, baking powder, and salt in a medium bowl. Whisk the agave, lemon juice, and vanilla extract together with the agar-agar mixture. Whisk the dry ingredients into the wet until a smooth batter forms, then fold in the strawberries.

3. Spoon the batter into the muffin pan, filling each cup about three-quarters full.

4. Bake for 18 to 22 minutes, until a knife inserted in the center comes out clean.

5. Remove from the oven, and let cool in the pan for 5 minutes. Transfer the cupcakes to a wire rack to cool completely before frosting with the whipped coconut cream.

GOITROGEN ALERT:
max 6 to 8 servings
per week

CHILLED STRAWBERRY CREAM PIE

This chilled strawberry cream pie is naturally sweet with a thick, creamy consistency and a bright pink color, baked into a flaky coconut flour crust. Not only are strawberries naturally sweet, but they are full of antioxidants as well as vitamin C, manganese, iodine, and dietary fiber.

Makes 8 to 10 servings

FOR THE CRUST

1 cup sifted coconut flour

1 teaspoon iodized salt

½ cup coconut oil

¼ cup pure maple syrup

FOR THE FILLING

1 (14-ounce) can coconut milk

2 tablespoons agar-agar flakes

2½ cups chopped fresh strawberries

¼ cup plus 2 tablespoons pure maple syrup

1 teaspoon vanilla extract

1. Preheat the oven to 325°F.

2. To make the crust, combine the coconut flour and salt in a medium bowl. Cut in the coconut oil with a fork or a pastry blender, until a crumbled mixture forms. Stir in the maple syrup until a dough forms. Press into the bottom and sides of a 9-inch glass pie plate. Bake for 4 to 6 minutes, until just browned. Remove from the oven, and set aside to cool.

3. To make the filling, heat the coconut milk in a small saucepan over medium heat. Whisk in the agar-agar flakes, and bring to a boil while stirring constantly. Reduce the heat, and simmer for 5 minutes, until the agar is completely dissolved, then remove from the heat and cool for 5 minutes. Place the strawberries, maple syrup, and vanilla extract in a food processor, and blend until smooth. Add the coconut milk mixture, and blend until thoroughly combined.

4. Pour the filling into the cooled pie crust, and spread it evenly. Chill in the refrigerator until set, about 6 hours. Serve cold.

GOITROGEN ALERT:
max 6 to 8 servings
per week

CLASSIC PUMPKIN PIE

Pumpkin pie is a traditional fall favorite, but you can enjoy it any time of year. Made with a simple coconut flour crust and a naturally sweet filling, you don't have to feel guilty about indulging in this tasty treat. **Makes** 8 to 10 servings

FOR THE CRUST

2 tablespoons melted coconut oil

2 tablespoons pure maple syrup

2 tablespoons agar-agar flakes

2 tablespoons warm water

¼ cup plus 2 tablespoons sifted coconut flour

pinch of iodized salt

FOR THE FILLING

2¾ cups pumpkin puree

¼–½ cup agave

¼ cup plus 2 tablespoons canned coconut milk

1 tablespoon melted coconut oil

2 tablespoons arrowroot powder

2 teaspoons pumpkin pie spice

¼ teaspoon iodized salt

1. Preheat the oven to 350°F.

2. To make the crust, whisk together the coconut oil and maple syrup in a medium bowl. In a small bowl, whisk together the agar-agar and warm water. Whisk the agar-agar mixture, coconut flour, and salt into the coconut oil mixture. Stir into a soft dough, and press into a 9-inch glass pie plate. Set aside.

3. To make the filling, combine the ingredients in a blender and blend until smooth. Spread the filling in the prepared pie crust, and cover the edges with foil.

4. Bake for 45 to 60 minutes, until the center is set. Remove the foil from the edges during the last 10 to 15 minutes of baking. Remove the pie from the oven, and let cool to room temperature, then chill overnight before serving.

CINNAMON APPLE COCONUT CRISP

This crisp is naturally sweetened with fresh apples and a hint of maple syrup. Enjoy it warm with a scoop of Vanilla Coconut Milk Ice Cream (page 195).

Makes 6 to 8 (1-cup) servings

1½ pounds Granny Smith apples, peeled and thinly sliced

2 tablespoons fresh lemon juice

2 tablespoons pure maple syrup

1 teaspoon ground cinnamon

1 cup unsweetened shredded coconut

⅓ cup sifted coconut flour

¼ cup coconut butter

¼ cup melted coconut oil

1 teaspoon vanilla extract

1. Preheat the oven to 350°F.

2. Toss the apples with the lemon juice, maple syrup, and cinnamon. Spread the mixture in an 8-inch square glass or ceramic baking dish.

3. In a medium bowl, combine the shredded coconut, coconut flour, coconut butter, coconut oil, and vanilla extract. Stir until thoroughly combined, and spread over the apple mixture.

4. Bake for 35 to 40 minutes, until the topping is browned and the apples are hot and bubbling. Remove from the oven, and let cool for 5 to 10 minutes before serving warm.

LEMON BLUEBERRY COBBLER

The sweetness of blueberries perfectly complements the tartness of lemon juice in this cobbler recipe, guaranteed to be a hit. Along with natural sweetness, the blueberries provide plenty of antioxidants.

Makes 8 to 10 (½-cup) servings

¼ cup agar-agar flakes

¼ cup warm water

½ cup sifted coconut flour

1 teaspoon baking soda

¼ teaspoon iodized salt

½ cup canned coconut milk

¼ cup melted coconut oil

¼ cup pure maple syrup

1½ teaspoons vanilla extract

4 cups fresh blueberries, rinsed well

¼ cup fresh lemon juice

1 tablespoon fresh lemon zest

1. Preheat the oven to 350°F, and grease an 8-inch square glass or ceramic baking dish with coconut oil.

2. To make the batter, whisk together the agar-agar flakes and warm water in a large bowl, and set aside. In a small bowl, whisk together the coconut flour, baking soda, and salt. Whisk the coconut milk, coconut oil, maple syrup, and vanilla extract into the agar-agar mixture. Add the dry ingredients to the wet ingredients, and whisk into a smooth batter.

3. In a large bowl, toss the blueberries with the lemon juice and lemon zest. Spread in the baking dish. Spoon the batter over the blueberries in large dollops, then spread evenly.

4. Bake for 30 to 35 minutes, until the topping is browned and the fruit is bubbling. Remove from the oven, and let cool for 5 to 10 minutes before serving warm.

PUMPKIN COCONUT DATE BALLS

This dessert is incredibly simple to prepare as it doesn't require cooking or baking. It's also healthy. In addition to being rich in dietary fiber as a gluten- and grain-free carbohydrate, pumpkin contains beta-carotene and a number of other powerful antioxidants. The dates contribute vitamin A, vitamin K, calcium, and folate while the coconut is rich in iron, manganese, and copper.

Makes about 24 (1-ball) servings

1 cup pitted Medjool dates	pinch of iodized salt
1 cup pumpkin puree	1 cup sifted coconut flour
1 tablespoon pure maple syrup	½–1 cup unsweetened shredded coconut

1. Place the dates in a food processor, and pulse until finely chopped. Add the pumpkin puree, maple syrup, and salt, and blend until smooth. Add the coconut flour, and blend until smooth and well combined.

2. Place the shredded coconut in a shallow bowl. Pinch off pieces of dough, and roll by hand into 1-inch balls. Roll each ball individually in the shredded coconut, and arrange them on a plate or baking sheet. Chill in the refrigerator until firm, then store in the refrigerator for up to 7 days.

COCONUT FLOUR
SHORTBREAD COOKIES

You don't have to give up shortbread cookies just because you're on the Hashimoto's diet. These cookies are just as simple to make and delicious to eat as standard shortbread cookies. To make the recipe vegan-friendly, substitute pure maple syrup or agave for the honey.

Makes about 2 dozen (1-cookie) servings

1 cup sifted coconut flour

¾ cups coconut oil

2–3 tablespoons raw honey

1 teaspoon vanilla extract

¼ teaspoon iodized salt

1. Preheat the oven to 350°F, and line two baking sheets with parchment paper.

2. Place the coconut flour in a large bowl, then cut in the coconut oil using a fork or pastry blender. Stir in the honey, vanilla extract and salt until a smooth dough forms.

3. Pinch off pieces of dough, and roll by hand into small balls. Place on the baking sheets, spacing at least 2 inches apart. Flatten to about ¼ inch thick using the tines of a fork.

4. Bake for 6 to 8 minutes, until the edges just start to brown.

5. Remove from the oven, but leave the cookies on the baking sheets to cool completely before serving.

SPICE COOKIES

If you aren't a fan of overly sweet desserts, these spice cookies might be right up your alley. Sweetened to taste with maple syrup and spiked with ginger and cloves, the cookies are loaded with flavor.

Makes 12 (1-cookie) servings

⅓ cup sifted coconut flour

¼ cup coconut oil

1–2 tablespoons pure maple syrup

½ teaspoon grated fresh ginger

¼ teaspoon ground cloves

pinch of freshly ground black pepper

pinch of iodized salt

1. Preheat the oven to 350°F, and line a baking sheet with parchment paper.

2. Whisk together the coconut flour, coconut oil, and maple syrup in a medium bowl. Stir in the ginger, cloves, black pepper, and salt until a smooth dough forms.

3. Pinch off pieces of dough, and roll by hand into 1-inch balls. Place on the baking sheet, spacing about 2 inches apart. Gently flatten about halfway with the palm of your hand.

4. Bake for 8 to 10 minutes, until golden brown. Remove from the oven, and leave on the baking sheet to cool completely before serving.

SWEET LEMON COOKIES

These have a crisp outer crust and a soft, lemon-flavored center. Prepare this recipe with Meyer lemons or, for an alternative flavor, try it with fresh orange juice and orange zest in place of lemon.

Makes about 36 (1-cookie) servings

1 tablespoon agar-agar flakes

1 tablespoon warm water

½ cup melted coconut oil

¼ cup canned coconut milk

¼ cup agave

1 tablespoon fresh lemon juice

1 teaspoon fresh lemon zest

1 cup sifted coconut flour

2 teaspoons baking powder

¼ teaspoon iodized salt

1. Whisk together the agar-agar and warm water in a small bowl then set aside.

2. Combine the coconut oil, coconut milk, and agave in a medium bowl. Whisk in the lemon juice, lemon zest, and the agar-agar mixture. In a separate medium bowl, whisk together the coconut flour, baking powder, and salt. Whisk the wet ingredients into the dry until thoroughly combined into a dough.

3. Roll the dough by hand into a ball, wrap in plastic, and chill in the refrigerator for 1 hour.

4. Preheat the oven to 350°F, and line two baking sheets with parchment paper.

5. Remove the dough from the refrigerator, and sandwich it between two pieces of parchment paper. Roll the dough ⅛ inch thick, and cut out the cookies using small cookie cutters. Place on the baking sheets, spacing about 1 inch apart.

6. Bake for 6 to 8 minutes, until the edges just begin to brown. Remove from the oven, and let cool completely on the baking sheets before serving.

EASY BANANA COOKIE BITES

These bites are an indulgent treat that are good for you! Enjoy them in a single bite, especially if you need a quick sampling of something sweet! Bananas are rich in potassium and a good source of iodine.

Makes 12 (3-cookie) servings

¼ cup plus 2 tablespoons sifted coconut flour

¼ teaspoon baking powder

pinch of iodized salt

1 small ripe banana, mashed

½ cup canned coconut milk

1 tablespoon raw honey or agave

1. Preheat the oven to 350°F, and line a baking sheet with parchment paper.

2. Whisk together the coconut flour, baking powder, and salt in a medium bowl. Stir in the banana, coconut milk, and honey or agave until fully combined.

3. Drop the cookie dough in rounded teaspoons on the baking sheet, spacing them about 1 inch apart. Gently flatten by pressing your thumb in the center of the cookie.

4. Bake for 8 to 10 minutes, until firm and just browned on the edges. Remove from the oven, and cool completely on a wire baking sheet before serving.

Conclusion

If you have been diagnosed with Hashimoto's disease, the weight and the stress of living with the condition may make you feel as though you are doing it alone. In reality, millions of people in the United States have Hashimoto's, and more are diagnosed every day. As the leading cause of hypothyroidism and one of the most common autoimmune diseases, Hashimoto's is the subject of a great deal of medical research. This is good news for you! While it is true that autoimmune diseases like Hashimoto's cannot be cured, there is absolutely no reason you cannot live a normal life with this condition.

Medical treatments for Hashimoto's disease have become more advanced in the past few decades, and synthetic hormone therapy has become the standard. Even if you are receiving medical treatment for your Hashimoto's, however, you may still be experiencing symptoms. If you are, your best plan is to make some healthy changes to your diet and your lifestyle. The Hashimoto's diet, as described in this book, is specifically designed to reduce or reverse many of the complications associated with Hashimoto's. By making healthy changes to your diet, you can reduce inflammation, rebalance your hormones, and heal your digestive system. After just a few short weeks on this diet, you may feel like a completely new person!

Hashimoto's disease is a serious condition, but it doesn't have to ruin your life. In fact, by following your prescribed treatment plan and switching to the Hashimoto's diet, you could actually go into remission. Hashimoto's disease may be something you have, but it doesn't have to become all that you are. If you are ready to break free from the confines of this condition and take back control of your health and your life, take to heart all of the tools and information provided in this book. The Hashimoto's diet may be the key to helping you rediscover who you were before Hashimoto's and who you want to be for the rest of your life.

Appendix A:
Autoimmune Diseases

"The immune system is composed of special cells and organs that deal with invaders and allergens. The cells create antibodies to fight off the infection or foreign intruders. To defend the body the immunity must recognize what is self or what belongs to the body and what is non-self or foreign to the body."

—Dr. Ananya Mandal, "What Is Autoimmune Disease?"[43]

Hashimoto's is one of the most common autoimmune diseases in addition to being one of the most common causes of hypothyroidism. If you have Hashimoto's disease, you may already have a thorough grasp of how the disease affects the body, particularly the thyroid gland. But if you are like the majority of Americans, your familiarity with autoimmune disease may be fairly limited. This is not a matter of being undereducated or ill-informed; the truth is that even most doctors and researchers still have a limited understanding about how autoimmune diseases develop. Learning more about autoimmune disease in general may help you to better understand the effects of Hashimoto's on the body, and it may also put into context the dietary recommendations for Hashimoto's management recommended in this book. This section provides an overview of autoimmune disease as well as information about common autoimmune diseases and their effects on the body.

OVERVIEW OF AUTOIMMUNE DISEASE

According to the American Autoimmune Related Disease Association (AARDA), autoimmune disease ranks among the top 10 leading causes of death in females, both children and women up to 64 years of age. Furthermore, an estimated 1 out of 12 men have some kind of autoimmune disease.[44] These numbers may shock you, but even more frightening is the fact that autoimmune disorders are becoming increasingly more common with each passing day. It is also true, however, that there are many clinical trials and research studies devoted to discovering more effective treatments for these diseases. New medical advancements are constantly being made in the fight against autoimmune disease. Hashimoto's disease is just one of the many autoimmune conditions known to affect millions of people around the world and it too is the subject of promising research.

The human body contains many types of cells, each with its own unique function. White blood cells (WBCs), also known as leukocytes, account for approximately 1 percent of blood, but they play an incredibly important role in the body. They are the soldiers of the immune system, constantly at war against bacteria, viruses, and other pathogens that threaten to invade the body and affect health.[45]

WBCs are produced in the bone marrow, and—because some types of these cells have very short lifespans—bone marrow is in constant production mode. Even though the body constantly produces WBCs, certain conditions can lead to a low WBC count, and a low count increases susceptibility to illness and infection. Autoimmune disease is one of the most common underlying factors that may contribute to a low count.[46]

When a potentially pathogenic material (antigen) enters the body, WBCs begin to produce antibodies—these are highly specialized proteins that correspond to a specific antigen. The antibodies bind themselves to the antigens and disable their harmful action. In the case of autoimmune disorders, the immune system is unable to distinguish between harmful antigens and the body's own tissue. As a result, the immune system begins to attack both. Autoimmune disorders can affect all types of cells, tissues, and organs, including red blood cells, blood vessels, endocrine glands, connective tissues, muscles, joints, and skin.[47]

Somewhere between 80 and 100 autoimmune disorders have been identified. Certain risk factors—such as sex, age, ethnicity, genetics, and various environmental factors—can impact a person's likelihood of developing one of these conditions. For example, a woman is at the greatest risk for developing an autoimmune condition during her reproductive years. Autoimmune diseases are also more common in younger people and in Latinos, Native Americans, and African Americans.

A family history of autoimmune disorders increases the risk,[48] and exposure to environmental agents including heavy metals, chemical pesticides, and certain medications such as hydralazine and procainamide may be a contributing factor as well. There is also some evidence to suggest that certain viral and bacterial infections increase a person's susceptibility to autoimmune disease, although more research needs to be conducted.

COMMON AUTOIMMUNE DISORDERS

While the National Institutes of Health estimates that nearly 24 million Americans are affected by some type of autoimmune disorder, AARDA suggests that the actual number is much greater—closer to 50 million.[49] Autoimmune diseases come in many forms, although the symptoms are similar. They may include fever, chronic fatigue, rashes, joint pain, and a general feeling of malaise. Dr. Datis Kharrazian, a chiropractor and alternative health practitioner, suggests that autoimmune disorders are progressive, going through three common stages: silent autoimmunity, autoimmune reactivity, and autoimmune disease.[50]

In the first stage of autoimmune disease, the immune system begins to attack the body's own healthy tissue but has yet to make a significant impact on the function of the body as a whole. Routine lab tests may show elevated antibody levels, but definitive symptoms are unlikely during this stage. As the disease progresses into the second stage, symptoms start to manifest. During this stage, the immune system begins to do actual damage to the target tissue, which results in significantly elevated antibody levels. It is during this stage that Hashimoto's patients are likely to display signs of impaired thyroid function.

During the third stage of autoimmune disease, significant destruction of the target tissue has already occurred to the point where it can be identified with an ultrasound or MRI. Diagnostic testing is likely to reveal elevated antibodies, loss of function in the affected organ or system, and dangerous side effects and symptoms such as severe anemia, hormone imbalance, and difficulty breathing. For Hashimoto's patients in this stage of the disease, the majority of the thyroid has been destroyed and the production of thyroid hormone has probably stopped completely, resulting in symptoms such as joint and muscle pain, increased sensitivity to cold, weight gain, and puffiness in the face.

Hashimoto's disease is just one of the many autoimmune diseases that have been identified and studied. Other common autoimmune disorders include the following:

ADDISON'S DISEASE—Another of the three most common autoimmune disorders, Addison's disease occurs when the adrenal glands fail to produce enough of three key hormones: glucocorticoid hormones (for example, cortisol), mineralocorticoid hormones (for example, aldosterone), and sex hormones. This disease can cause changes in the appearance of the skin as well as dizziness, weakness, chronic diarrhea, and weight loss.

CELIAC SPRUE DISEASE—Also known as celiac disease, this condition occurs when the body produces an autoimmune response in reaction to eating gluten. It causes chronic inflammation and damage to the lining of the small intestine, which can lead to weight loss, abdominal pain, gas and bloating, constipation, lactose intolerance, and changes in bowel movements.

DIABETES (TYPE 1)—Frequently cited as one of the most common autoimmune diseases, type 1 diabetes occurs when the body is unable to produce adequate insulin. It leads to high blood sugar levels, causing symptoms such as chronic fatigue, frequent hunger and thirst, blurred vision, numbness in the feet, and increased urination. The condition can manifest at any age.

GRAVES' DISEASE—This condition is another autoimmune disease that affects the thyroid. In contrast to Hashimoto's disease, Graves' disease causes hyperthyroidism (over-activity of the thyroid gland). Some of the most common symptoms of this condition include anxiety and irritability, unexplained weight loss, heart palpitations, tremors, bulging eyes, and thickened skin on the shins or feet.

INFLAMMATORY BOWEL DISEASE—This autoimmune condition causes chronic inflammation to part or all of the digestive system. IBD is actually a category of conditions that includes Crohn's disease, ulcerative colitis, and collagenous colitis. IBD generally causes digestive symptoms, such as abdominal pain and cramping, constipation and diarrhea as well as chronic fatigue, joint pain, and rectal bleeding.

MULTIPLE SCLEROSIS—Commonly known as MS, this degenerative autoimmune disorder affects the brain and spinal cord. Damage to the myelin sheaths protecting the nerves in the central nervous system leads to nerve damage and impaired function. Some of the most common symptoms of MS are fatigue, weakness or numbness in the body and extremities, difficulty walking, vertigo, bladder and bowel problems, emotional changes, and, in some cases, seizures or tremors.

PERNICIOUS ANEMIA—Anemia is a condition characterized by low red blood cell count. Pernicious anemia occurs when the ability of the intestines to absorb vitamin B12 is impaired, leading to a decrease in red blood cell production. Vitamin B12 deficiency generally causes symptoms such as weakness, fatigue, tingling or numbness in the extremities, headaches, and chest pains.

PSORIASIS—A type of skin disorder, psoriasis causes skin cells to multiply up to 10 times faster than normal, prompting a layer of dead skin cells to form on the surface. Psoriasis can lead to redness and irritated skin as well as scaly lesions and pitting of the nails.

RHEUMATOID ARTHRITIS—One of the three most common autoimmune diseases, rheumatoid arthritis involves chronic inflammation of the joints and surrounding tissues, and sometimes bone and joint deformities. This condition typically affects the joints in the wrists, fingers, knees, ankles, and feet. It is a progressive disease that worsens over time.

SJÖGREN'S SYNDROME — This autoimmune disease primarily affects the salivary glands and the glands that produce tears, but it can also affect the lungs and kidneys as well as other body parts. Dry mouth and dry eyes are two of the most common symptoms of Sjögren's Syndrome, but other symptoms may include joint pain, skin rashes, persistent cough, and chronic fatigue.

SYSTEMIC LUPUS ERYTHEMATOSUS — More commonly known as lupus, this autoimmune disease occurs when the body mistakenly attacks and destroys healthy tissue in the skin, joints, brain, kidneys, and other organs. It can cause joint pain and swelling as well as chronic fatigue, unexplained fever, hair loss, and other symptoms that correlate with the part of the body affected by the disease.

VITILIGO — This disease causes the skin to lose color, or pigment. It can affect the skin on any part of the body as well as hair color and eye color. The rate and extent of depigmentation is unpredictable.

DIAGNOSING AN AUTOIMMUNE DISEASE

The methods for diagnosing autoimmune diseases vary from one disease to another. Diagnostic tests may include complete blood count (CBC), autoantibody tests, C-reactive protein (CRP) tests, comprehensive metabolic panel, and urinalysis in addition to a complete physical exam. Autoimmune diseases cannot be cured, but in most cases they can be managed. Treatment options for these disorders are generally aimed at reducing symptoms, controlling the autoimmune process, and rebuilding the immune system. Autoimmune disorders are chronic (long lasting) but, with proper treatment, they can go into remission, sometimes for years at a time.[51]

EFFECTS OF AUTOIMMUNE DISEASE ON THE BODY

Different autoimmune disorders affect the body in different ways, depending on the tissue targeted in the attack. Many different parts of the body, including cells, glands, tissues, muscles, joints, and skin, can be affected.[52] Some of the most common symptoms of autoimmune disease include chronic fatigue, fever, and general malaise. Symptoms may decline or disappear entirely during periods of remission, and they can worsen significantly during flare-ups.

In addition to these general symptoms, autoimmune disease can have some devastating long-term effects on the body, such as chronic inflammation, hormone imbalance, and damage to the digestive system.

CHRONIC INFLAMMATION

Inflammation is the body's response to injury or infection. The body sends extra blood to the site to start the healing process—this is what produces the redness and swelling that develops following an injury. Acute inflammation lasts for only a few days, but chronic inflammation can last for months and may not be outwardly visible. When an autoimmune disease causes the immune system to attack healthy cells and tissue, inflammation is often the first symptom to develop. It commonly triggers the body to produce high levels of chemokines and cytokines, which lead to chronic inflammation in the affected tissues. In addition to the devastating effects of autoimmune disease, chronic inflammation alone can be very damaging to the body.

According to Dr. Isaac Eliaz, a holistic medicine practitioner and integrative medical doctor, the inflammatory process "creates a type of heat and friction on a physiological level, similar to rubbing fabric together—eventually [the fabric] begins to degrade." This degradation causes changes in cellular function, often leading to abnormalities in the healing process. Chronic inflammation can also have an effect on internal organs, and it has been linked to skin problems, musculoskeletal issues, mood disorders, and mental imbalances.[53]

HORMONE IMBALANCE

Certain autoimmune disorders, like Hashimoto's, target various hormone-producing glands in the body. As these glands become more and more damaged, their ability to produce vital hormones is impaired, which leads to hormone imbalance. Adrenal glands are responsible for producing the hormones—cortisol testosterone, progesterone, DHEA, and epinephrine—that regulate metabolic function. Cortisol is particularly important because it helps to regulate the immune system. Cortisol levels that are too high or too low can cause chronic inflammation, frequent infections, and an increased risk for other autoimmune diseases.

Autoimmune diseases that affect the thyroid (Hashimoto's and Graves') can impair the body's ability to respond to viruses and to combat inflammation. Abnormal estrogen levels have also been linked to thyroid problems and impaired immunity. Hormone imbalance in general can have some very serious side effects, including chronic fatigue, poor sleep quality, chronic stress, impaired immune system, and changes in weight. Imbalanced hormone levels can also contribute to mood swings, chronic inflammation, unexplained pain, chronic illness, and mental problems such as memory issues and difficulty concentrating.[54]

GUT DAMAGE

The digestive system is very complex, and its function is tied directly to the function of other important systems in the body. In fact, about 80 percent of the immune system is located in the gut, so it's not surprising that impaired immune function or an overactive immune system is linked to gut damage.[55] Dr. Alessio Fasano, pediatric gastroenterologist and founder of the University of Maryland Center for Celiac Research, suggests that all autoimmune diseases have three things in common: "a genetic susceptibility, antigen exposure, and increased intestinal permeability."[56] Genetic susceptibility simply refers to a family history of autoimmune disease, and antigen exposure describes the autoimmune activity that causes the symptoms. Increased intestinal permeability refers to the intestine being porous enough that harmful substances can pass through the walls and into the bloodstream.

The main purpose of the digestive system is to process food and extract nutrients. To do its job properly, the intestines must exhibit some degree of permeability to allow nutrients to pass into the bloodstream. While some degree of permeability is important and healthy, too much permeability allows potentially harmful substances to pass through. This increased intestinal permeability, also known as leaky gut syndrome, is widely considered to be a significant factor in the development of serious conditions like Crohn's disease, celiac disease, chronic giardiasis, atopic eczema, and even alcoholism. Leaky gut syndrome can also lead to malnutrition, the spread of infection, and food sensitivities and intolerances.[57]

Appendix B:
Exercise and Hashimoto's Disease

"HIIT [high-intensity interval training] forces your heart and body to learn how to adapt to constantly changing conditions. It also kicks the metabolism into high gear, which continues for hours after the workout in a sort of 'after-burn' effect called EPOC, or Excess Post-exercise Oxygen Consumption,... Other than [increasing] caloric output, HIIT also helps modulate insulin resistance, reduce abdominal fat, reduce oxidative stress, and improve antioxidant status."

—Susan Vennerholm, *Autoimmune Paleo*[58]

Many people with Hashimoto's disease suffer from chronic fatigue. When you feel tired and run down all the time, you may find it difficult to motivate yourself to leave the house, let alone get some exercise. However, exercise is highly beneficial as a supplemental therapy for autoimmune diseases like Hashimoto's.

Before you hit the gym, take the time to learn about the *right* kind of exercise for Hashimoto's. If you aren't careful and you overexert yourself, you could end up making things worse. Overexertion can lead to a spike in cortisol production, which can increase your risk for digestive problems, mood issues, and more exhaustion. The stress that overexercising puts on the body can have a negative impact on the hypothalamic-pituitary-adrenalaxis (HPA), which plays a role in regulating both thyroid and adrenal function. The stress can also exacerbate leaky gut problems.[59]

SO WHAT KIND OF EXERCISE IS BEST FOR HASHIMOTO'S DISEASE?

HIIT, or high-intensity interval training, is the best choice because it can be accomplished in 30 minutes or less, which limits the amount of stress you put on your body—it also burns more calories than other types of exercise performed for the same amount of time. The term "high-intensity" means expending the maximum amount of effort over short intervals. Rather than walking briskly for an hour or running on the treadmill at a steady pace for 30 minutes, you alternate between periods of maximum-intensity and low-intensity exercise for a total of just 20 minutes or so. Of course, HIIT is not for everyone. If you suffer from muscle aches, joint pain, or swelling due to Hashimoto's you can adjust the intensity of your workout to suit your abilities. If you are limited to walking, you can still perform HIIT by alternating between periods of fast walking and slow walking. You could also alternate between periods of walking on an incline and walking flat.

If you've never tried HIIT, you may be skeptical about the benefits of a workout program that can be completed in such a limited time. What you need to understand is that with this type of workout the focus is not on time but on intensity. High-intensity exercise can stimulate significant changes in the body at the biochemical level.[60] Some of the most important potential benefits of HIIT include:

- Balancing hormone levels

- Restoring the body's natural sensitivity to insulin

- Increasing the natural production of human growth hormone (HGH) to boost metabolism

- Building lean muscle mass

- Burning more calories than any other exercise over the same time period

The beauty of HIIT is that you can customize your workout according to your preferences and limitations. If you have bad knees and can't run on a treadmill, you can use an exercise bike instead. If you don't like the idea of running or cycling, you can do bodyweight exercises like push-ups or strength-building exercises like jumping jacks instead. In the end, it doesn't really matter what kind of exercise you do as long as you alternate between periods of maximum exertion and rest. Just be sure to perform the exercises only as quickly as you can with proper form, to avoid injuring yourself.

To give you a better idea of what a HIIT workout looks like, try one of the following workout plans.

1 round = 40 seconds for each exercise
(30-second work followed by 10-second rest)

Do 3 rounds; rest for 1 minute between rounds

1. Jab, Cross, Kick (left side)	Stand in boxer's stance with your right foot positioned in front of your left foot with your hips cocked to the right and your weight on your back heel. Hold your fists in front of your face in a boxing position, then jab forward with your left fist, cross punch with your right fist, and kick forward with your right foot. Repeat as quickly as possible.
2. Jab, Cross, Kick (right side)	Stand in boxer's stance with your left foot positioned in front of your right foot with your hips cocked to the left and your weight on your back heel. Hold your fists in front of your face in a boxing position, then jab forward with your right fist, cross punch with your left fist, and kick forward with your left foot. Repeat as quickly as possible.
3. Jumping Jacks	Stand upright with your feet hip-width apart and your arms hanging down at your sides. Jump and thrust your feet out while raising your arms above your heart, then thrust your feet back together while lowering your arms. Repeat as quickly as possible.
4. Sumo Squats	Stand upright with your feet shoulder-width apart, your toes pointed outward at a 45-degree angle, and your weight on your heels. Thrust your hips back as if you were sitting in a chair, preserving the natural arch in your back, and lower yourself until your thighs are parallel to the floor. Tighten your abs, quads, and glutes, then push back on your heels and return to the starting position. Repeat as quickly as possible.

1 round = 1 minute for each exercise
(45-second work followed by 15-second rest)

Do 3 rounds; rest for 1 minute between rounds

1. Push-Ups	Hold your body up off the ground with your legs straight and your hands positioned just below your shoulders. Lower to the ground, keeping your body straight, until your chest is a few inches from the floor. Push yourself back up into the starting position, and repeat as quickly as possible. If you cannot perform regular push-ups with good form for an entire minute, drop to your knees instead of your toes, but make an effort to keep your core tight and your back straight.
2. Squats	Stand upright with your feet shoulder-width apart, your toes pointed forward, and your weight on your heels. Thrust your hips back as if you were sitting in a chair, preserving the natural arch in your back, and lower yourself until your thighs are parallel to the floor. Tighten your abs, quads, and glutes, then push back on your heels and return to the starting position. Repeat as quickly as possible.
3. Butt Kicks	Stand upright, then jog or walk in place, kicking your left heel up behind you to touch your backside, if you can. Repeat with the right leg, alternating as quickly as possible.
4. Triceps Dips	Sit on the edge of a chair with your hands on either side of your body, gripping the edge of the chair. Scoot yourself out so your bottom is no longer touching the chair then lower your bottom to the ground by bending at the elbow. Lower yourself as far as you can, then press back up. Repeat as quickly as possible.
5. Side Lunges	Stand upright with your feet together, toes facing forward, and your weight on your heels. Step out to the left, bending your left knee at a 90-degree angle in a deep lunge, making sure your knee doesn't bend past your toes and keeping your right leg straight. Then push up with your foot to return to the starting position. Repeat with the right leg, and alternate as quickly as possible.

ADVANCED LEVEL—25-MINUTE WORKOUT

1 round = 20 seconds exercise A then 20 seconds exercise B in the order listed followed by 20 seconds rest

Do 4 rounds; rest for 1 minute between rounds

1A. Squat Jacks	Hold your hands behind your head, and stand with your feet hip-width apart. Thrust your hips back and bend your knees, lowering yourself until your thighs are parallel to the ground. Push off the ground with your heels, maintaining a squat position, and open your legs into a wide stance. Jump back into the start position and repeat as quickly as possible, never breaking the squat.
1B. Push-Ups with Oblique Knees	Start in a plank position with your hands positioned under your shoulders and your weight supported by your toes. Bring your right knee in toward your right elbow, return to start, bring it in toward your left elbow, and return to start. Perform a push-up, then repeat on the opposite side and keep alternating.
2A. Star Jumps	Stand with your feet hip-width apart and your arms hanging down at your side. Squat down, then push off the ground with your feet, raising your arms above your head and spreading your legs wide (your body should form a star shape). Bring your arms and legs back down as you descend and land in the starting position then repeat as quickly as possible.
2B. Mountain Climbers	Start in a plank position with your hands positioned under your shoulders and your weight supported by your toes. Bring your right knee in toward your right elbow, then return to start. Bring your left knee toward your left elbow, then return to start. Repeat as quickly as possible, keeping your back straight.
3A. Squat Jumps	Start with your feet shoulder-width apart, then thrust your hips back and bend your knees, lowering yourself until your thighs are parallel to the ground. When you reach parallel, push off the ground with your heels and jump, then return to the start position and repeat as quickly as possible.
3B. Speed Skaters	Stand with your feet shoulder-width apart, then step out with your right leg and lunge, reaching your left hand toward your right foot. Hop your right leg back to the middle, then step out with your left leg and reach with your right hand. Repeat as quickly as possible.

4A. High Knees	Stand with your feet hip-width apart and your arms hanging at your sides. Jump from one foot to the other, raising your knee as high as you can each time (try to reach at least hip height), repeating as quickly as possible.
4B. Jumping Lunges	Stand with your feet hip-width apart, then step forward with your right leg and lunge until your left knee brushes the ground. Push off the ground with your front leg and jump, switching legs in the air. Cushion your landing, lunge with the opposite leg, and repeat as quickly as possible.

30-MINUTE TREADMILL OR EXERCISE BIKE WORKOUT

If you are using a treadmill, set the incline to 1.5 for the duration of the workout. If you are using a stationary bike, choose a level of resistance that you can maintain for the entire duration.

MINUTES	SPEED (MPH)
0–4:00	4.0
4:00–4:30	5.5
4:30–5:00	8
5:00–5:30	5.5
5:30–6:00	8
6:00–6:30	5.5
6:30–7:00	8
7:00–7:30	5.5
7:30–8:00	8
8:00–8:30	5.5
8:30–9:00	8
9:00–14:00	6
14:00–19:00	repeat minutes 4–9
19:00–24:00	repeat minutes 9–14
24:00–28:00	6.5
28:00–30:00	3.5

Appendix C:
Glossary of Important Terms

Adrenal gland—An endocrine gland responsible for producing various hormones including adrenaline, aldosterone, and cortisol.

Animal thyroid extract—A natural thyroid supplement taken from the thyroid gland of an animal (usually a pig).

Antibody—A highly specialized protein produced by the immune system that corresponds to a specific antigen.

Antigen—Any potentially pathogenic material that enters the body.

Anti-thyroid microsomal antibody test—A test used to determine whether anti-thyroid antibodies are present; frequently used to confirm a diagnosis of Hashimoto's disease.

Autoimmune disease—A condition in which the immune system mistakenly identifies its own healthy tissue as an antigen and works to destroy it.

Autoimmune protocol (AIP)—A Paleo, gluten-free diet designed to address problems with inflammation and gut damage, especially when these problems are caused by autoimmune disease.

Central nervous system—A division of the human nervous system; consists of the nerves, the spinal cord, and the brain.

Endocrine system—A network of glands and organs responsible for producing the hormones that help to regulate metabolism, tissue function, growth and development, reproduction, mood, and sleep.

Fermentation—The chemical breakdown of foods by bacteria, yeast, or other organisms; the process used to create alcoholic beverages; a method of natural food preservation that increases the nutritional value of the ingredients.

Free-radical damage—Damage to the structure, DNA or membranes of cells caused by free radicals—highly reactive atoms or molecules, which contain unpaired electrons, allowing them to "steal" electrons from cells.

Gland—A specialized organ that filters certain materials or substances from the blood and processes them, secreting the finished product back into the bloodstream for use throughout the body.

Goiter—A swelling that forms on the front or side of the neck; often one of the first signs of Hashimoto's disease or hypothyroidism.

Goitrogen—A substance found in certain foods (for example, broccoli, cauliflower, kale, peaches, spinach, and strawberries) that can impair the ability of the thyroid to produce thyroid hormones.

Hashimoto's thyroiditis—A condition characterized by inflammation and destruction of the thyroid gland; the most common cause of hypothyroidism.

Human chorionic gonadotropin (hCG)—A hormone produced in the placenta that stimulates the thyroid gland to produce more thyroid hormone, particularly during pregnancy.

Hyperthyroidism—An overactive thyroid gland.

Hypothyroidism—An underactive thyroid gland.

Increased intestinal permeability—A condition in which the lining of the intestine becomes abnormally permeable, allowing food products and harmful substances to leak into the body; also called leaky gut syndrome.

Inflammation—The body's natural response to injury or trauma; chronic inflammation is often the result of autoimmune disease.

Leaky gut syndrome—See Increased intestinal permeability.

Leukocytes—White blood cells (WBCs); the active cells of the immune system that work to destroy harmful bacteria, viruses, and other pathogens.

Metabolism—A term used to describe the chemical and biological reactions that take place in the human body in order to sustain life.

Myxedema—A complication of hypothyroidism that may cause increased sensitivity to cold, drowsiness, and lethargy, often followed eventually by unconsciousness.

Nightshade—A family of plants that is known to cause inflammation and may also contribute to intestinal permeability and autoimmune disease; examples include tomatoes, potatoes, eggplant, peppers, and tomatillos, and certain spices including paprika, cayenne, and chili powder.

Oxidative stress—An imbalance in the production of free radicals and the body's ability to counteract or detoxify their harmful effects. Oxidative stress may contribute to the development of serious health problems including Alzheimer's disease, cancer, and Parkinson's disease.

Paleo diet—A diet that does not include any foods that would not have been readily available to our Paleolithic ancestors; excludes grains, legumes, dairy products, artificial sweeteners, and processed foods.

Peripheral nervous system—One division of the human nervous system; consists of sensory and motor neurons, which send and receive signals from the central nervous system.

Pituitary gland—The gland responsible for controlling growth and development; also plays a role in supporting the function of other endocrine glands.

Probiotic—Beneficial bacteria that help to support the digestive system.

Reverse T3—An inactive form of the T3 hormone; a metabolite of the T4 hormone produced through the conversion of T4 that is incapable of delivering oxygen or energy to the cells.

Stealth infection—An infection that cannot be detected by routine lab tests.

Synthetic thyroid supplement—A manufactured thyroid hormone supplement; the most common type of thyroid replacement therapy as a treatment for Hashimoto's disease.

Thyroid gland—The butterfly-shaped endocrine gland that is located in the lower front of the neck. Responsible for producing thyroid hormones and for helping the body to utilize energy efficiently by regulating body temperature and maintaining the healthy function of the heart, brain, muscles, and other organs.

Thyroid hormone replacement therapy—The most common treatment for Hashimoto's disease; uses synthetic or natural thyroid hormone supplements to simulate or restore healthy thyroid function.

Thyroid lymphoma—A potential complication of hypothyroidism; a type of thyroid cancer.

Thyroid stimulating hormone (TSH)—A hormone produced by the pituitary gland that activates thyroid hormones.

Thyroiditis—Inflammation of the thyroid gland.

Thyroxine (T4)—Known as a prohormone; has minimal hormonal effect itself, but can amplify the effects of the active hormone, triiodothyronine.

Triiodothyronine (T3)—The active form of the thyroid hormone; about 20 percent of the body's supply is secreted directly into the bloodstream from the thyroid gland itself.

TSH Test—A test to determine the amount of TSH being produced by the pituitary gland; the first blood test typically ordered to confirm a diagnosis of Hashimoto's disease.

T3 test—A blood test used to determine the amount of T3 in the blood; frequently used as a method for diagnosing Hashimoto's disease.

T4 test—A blood test to determine the amount of T4 in the blood; frequently used as a method for diagnosing Hashimoto's disease.

Vegan—Someone who chooses to abstain from the consumption of all animal products including eggs, dairy, and honey.

Vegetarian—Someone who chooses to abstain from the consumption of meat products; some vegetarians eat eggs and dairy products.

ENDNOTES

1 Marc Ryan, "Hashimoto's Is an Autoimmune Disease, So Why Is Everyone Ignoring the Autoimmune Part?" Hashimoto's Healing, accessed May 15, 2016, www.hashimotoshealing.com/hashimotos-is-an-autoimmune-disease-so-why-is-everyone-ignoring-the-autoimmune-part.

2 "Hashimoto's Disease," National Institute of Diabetes and Digestive and Kidney Diseases, accessed May 15, 2016, www.niddk.nih.gov/health-information/health-topics/endocrine/hashimotos-disease/Pages/fact-sheet.aspx.

3 Jen Sinkler, "Easing Out of Hashimoto's," Thrive with Jen Sinkler, accessed May 15, 2016, www.jensinkler.com/easing-out-of-hashimoto-thyroid.

4 "Hashimoto's Disease," Mayo Clinic, accessed May 15, 2016, www.mayoclinic.org/diseases-conditions/hashimotos-disease/basics/definition/con-20030293.

5 Julie Roddick, "Autoimmune Disease," Healthline, accessed May 15, 2016, www.healthline.com/health/autoimmune-disorders#Overview1.

6 Michael Lam, "Post Bacteria and Post Viral Fatigue Syndrome in Adrenal Fatigue Syndrome," Dr. Lam, accessed May 15, 2016, www.drlam.com/blog/post-bacterial-and-post-viral-fatigue-in-adrenal-fatigue-syndrome/5500.

7 "Hashimoto's Disease," National Institute of Diabetes and Digestive and Kidney Diseases, accessed May 15, 2016, www.niddk.nih.gov/health-information/health-topics/endocrine/hashimotos-disease/Pages/fact-sheet.aspx.

8 Kresimira Milas, "Hashimoto's Thyroiditis Overview," Endocrine Web, accessed May 15, 2016, www.endocrineweb.com/conditions/hashimotos-thyroiditis/hashimotos-thyroiditis-overview/.

9 "Eating with Hashimoto's Disease," The Science of Eating, accessed May 15, 2016, http://thescienceofeating.com/food-combining-how-it-works/eating-with-hashimotos-disease.

10 "Hashimoto's Disease," National Institute of Diabetes and Digestive and Kidney Diseases, accessed May 15, 2016, www.niddk.nih.gov/health-information/health-topics/endocrine/hashimotos-disease/Pages/fact-sheet.aspx.

11 "Hashimoto's Disease," Mayo Clinic, accessed May 15, 2016, www.mayoclinic.org/diseases-conditions/hashimotos-disease/basics/definition/con-20030293.

12 James Norman, "Hypothyroidism: Too Little Thyroid Hormone," Endocrine Web, accessed May 15, 2016, www.endocrineweb.com/conditions/thyroid/hypothyroidism-too-little-thyroid-hormone.

13 Kim Ann Zimmerman, "Endocrine System: Facts, Functions and Diseases," LiveScience, accessed May 15, 2016, www.livescience.com/26496-endocrine-system.html.

14 "Triiodothryonine," You & Your Hormones, accessed May 15, 2016, www
    .yourhormones.info/Hormones/Triiodothyronine.aspx.

15 "Thyroid Information," American Thyroid Association, accessed May 15,
    2016, www.thyroid.org/thyroid-information.

16 "Hashimoto's Disease," National Institute of Diabetes and Digestive and
    Kidney Diseases, accessed May 15, 2016, www.niddk.nih.gov/health-
    information/health-topics/endocrine/hashimotos-disease/Pages/fact-
    sheet.aspx.

17 Eren Berber, "Complications of Hypothyroidism," Endocrine Web, accessed
    May 15, 2016, www.endocrineweb.com/conditions/hypothyroidism/
    complications-hypothyroidism.

18 "Hashimoto's Disease," National Institute of Diabetes and Digestive and
    Kidney Diseases, accessed May 15, 2016, www.niddk.nih.gov/health-
    information/health-topics/endocrine/hashimotos-disease/Pages/fact-
    sheet.aspx.

19 "Pregnancy and Thyroid Disease," National Institute of Diabetes and
    Digestive and Kidney Diseases, accessed May 15, 2016, www.niddk.nih
    .gov/health-information/health-topics/endocrine/pregnancy-and-
    thyroid-disease/Pages/fact-sheet.aspx.

20 Nikolas Robert Hedberg, *The Thyroid Alternative* (Renew Your Health,
    2011).

21 "TSH Test," Medline Plus, accessed July 5, 2016, www.nlm.nih.gov/
    medlineplus/ency/article/003684.htm.

22 "Hashimoto's Disease," National Institute of Diabetes and Digestive and
    Kidney Diseases, accessed May 15, 2016, www.niddk.nih.gov/health-
    information/health-topics/endocrine/hashimotos-disease/Pages/fact-
    sheet.aspx.

23 Kresimira Milas, "Hashimoto's Thyroiditis Overview," Endocrine Web,
    accessed May 15, 2016, www.endocrineweb.com/conditions/hashimotos-
    thyroiditis/hashimotos-thyroiditis-overview/.

24 Eren Berber, "What Is Thyroid Hormone Replacement Therapy?"
    Endocrine Web, accessed May 10, 2016, www.endocrineweb.com/
    conditions/hypothyroidism/what-thyroid-hormone-replacement-therapy.

25 Ibid.

26 Ibid.

27 Westin Childs, *Hashimoto's Diet Guide: How to Heal Your Thyroid and
    Boost Your Metabolism with the Thyroid Reset Diet* (Amazon Digital
    Services, 2015), Kindle edition.

28 "How to Boost Your Immune System," Harvard Health Publications,
    accessed May 15, 2016, www.health.harvard.edu/staying-healthy/how-to-
    boost-your-immune-system.

29 "5 Essential Supplements for Optimal Thyroid Health," Natural Endocrine
    Solutions, accessed May 15, 2016, www.naturalendocrinesolutions.com/
    articles/5-essential-supplements-optimal-thyroid-health.

30 "How to Boost Your Immune System." Harvard Health Publications, accessed May 15, 2016, www.health.harvard.edu/staying-healthy/how-to-boost-your-immune-system.

31 Westin Childs, *Hashimoto's Diet Guide: How to Heal Your Thyroid and Boost Your Metabolism with the Thyroid Reset Diet* (Amazon Digital Services, 2015), Kindle edition.

32 "How to Boost Your Immune System," Harvard Health Publications, accessed May 15, 2016, www.health.harvard.edu/staying-healthy/how-to-boost-your-immune-system.

33 Nikolas Hedberg and Danielle Cook, *The Complete Thyroid Health and Diet Guide: Understanding and Managing Thyroid Disease* (Toronto, ON: Robert Rose, 2015).

34 Karen Frazier, *The Hashimoto's Cookbook and Action Plan: 31 Days to Eliminate Toxins and Restore Thyroid Health through Diet* (Berkeley, CA: Rockridge Press, 2015).

35 *The Autoimmune Paleo Cookbook & Action Plan: A Practical Guide to Easing Your Autoimmune Disease Symptoms with Nourishing Food* (Berkeley, CA: Rockridge Press, 2015).

36 "What Are Phytonutrients?" Fruits & Veggies More Matters, accessed May 15, 2016, www.fruitsandveggiesmorematters.org/what-are-phytochemicals.

37 Karen Frazier, *The Hashimoto's Cookbook and Action Plan: 31 Days to Eliminate Toxins and Restore Thyroid Health through Diet* (Berkeley, CA: Rockridge Press, 2015).

38 Ibid.

39 Marcelle Pick, "Goitrogens and Thyroid Health—The Good News!" Women to Women, accessed May 15, 2016, www.womentowomen.com/thyroid-health/goitrogens-and-thyroid-health-the-good-news.

40 Westin Childs, *Hashimoto's Diet Guide: How to Heal Your Thyroid and Boost Your Metabolism with the Thyroid Reset Diet* (Amazon Digital Services, 2015), Kindle edition.

41 Kelly Torrens, "The Truth about Low-Fat Foods," BBC Good Food, accessed May 15, 2016, www.bbcgoodfood.com/howto/guide/truth-about-low-fat-foods.

42 Bec Mills, "Concept of Stealth Infections," Beyond the Bandaid, accessed May 15, 2016, http://beyondthebandaid.com.au/concept-of-stealth-infections.

43 Ananya Mandal, "What Is Autoimmune Disease?" News Medical, accessed June 11, 2016, www.news-medical.net/health/What-is-Autoimmune-Disease.aspx.

44 Marc Ryan, "Hashimoto's Is an Autoimmune Disease, So Why Is Everyone Ignoring the Autoimmune Part?" Hashimoto's Healing, accessed May 15, 2016, www.hashimotoshealing.com/hashimotos-is-an-autoimmune-disease-so-why-is-everyone-ignoring-the-autoimmune-part.

45 Judith Berry and Adam Levy, "What Are White Blood Cells?" University of
    Rochester Medical Center, accessed May 15, 2016, www.urmc.rochester
    .edu/encyclopedia/content.aspx?ContentTypeID=160&ContentID=35.

46 Valencia Higuera, "WBC (White Blood Cell) Count," Healthline, accessed
    May 15, 2016, www.healthline.com/health/wbc-count#TestResults5.

47 Kresimira Milas, "Hashimoto's Thyroiditis Overview," Endocrine Web,
    accessed May 15, 2016, www.endocrineweb.com/conditions/hashimotos-
    thyroiditis/hashimotos-thyroiditis-overview.

48 Judith Berry and Adam Levy, "What Are White Blood Cells?" University of
    Rochester Medical Center, accessed May 15, 2016, www.urmc.rochester
    .edu/encyclopedia/content.aspx?ContentTypeID=160&ContentID=35.

49 Marc Ryan, "Hashimoto's Is an Autoimmune Disease, So Why Is Everyone
    Ignoring the Autoimmune Part?" Hashimoto's Healing, accessed May 15,
    2016, www.hashimotoshealing.com/hashimotos-is-an-autoimmune-
    disease-so-why-is-everyone-ignoring-the-autoimmune-part.

50 Ibid.

51 Kresimira Milas, "Hashimoto's Thyroiditis Overview," Endocrine Web,
    accessed May 15, 2016, www.endocrineweb.com/conditions/hashimotos-
    thyroiditis/hashimotos-thyroiditis-overview.

52 Julie Roddick, "Autoimmune Disease," Healthline, accessed May 15, 2016,
    www.healthline.com/health/autoimmune-disorders.

53 "Doctor Speaks on Health Effects of Chronic Inflammation," News Medical,
    accessed May 15, 2016, www.news-medical.net/news/20110217/Doctor-
    speaks-on-health-effects-of-chronic-inflammation.aspx.

54 "TSH Test," Medline Plus, accessed July 5, 2016, www.nlm.nih.gov/
    medlineplus/ency/article/003684.htm.

55 Amy Myers, *The Autoimmune Solution: Prevent and Reverse the Full
    Spectrum of Inflammatory Symptoms and Diseases* (New York: Harper
    Collins, 2015).

56 Aglaée Jacob, "Gut Health and Autoimmune Disease," *Today's Dietitian*
    15, no. 2 (2013): 38, accessed May 15, 2016, www.todaysdietitian.com/
    newarchives/021313p38.shtml.

57 Simon Martin, "Intestinal Permeability," *BioMed Newsletter*, no. 11 (May
    1995), accessed May 15, 2016, www.anapsid.org/CND/diffdx/leakygut2
    .html.

58 Susan Vennerholm, "Cardio, High Intensity and Resistance Workouts:
    Which Is for Me?" Autoimmune-Paleo, accessed May 15, 2016, http://
    autoimmune-paleo.com/cardio-high-intensity-resistance-workouts-
    which-is-for-me.

59 Ibid.

60 Westin Childs, *Hashimoto's Diet Guide: How to Heal Your Thyroid and
    Boost Your Metabolism with the Thyroid Reset Diet* (Amazon Digital
    Services, 2015), Kindle edition.

RESOURCES

"5 Essential Supplements for Optimal Thyroid Health." Natural Endocrine Solutions. Accessed May 15, 2016. www .naturalendocrinesolutions.com/articles/5-essential-supplements-optimal-thyroid-health.

The Autoimmune Paleo Cookbook & Action Plan: A Practical Guide to Easing Your Autoimmune Disease Symptoms with Nourishing Food. Berkeley, CA: Rockridge Press, 2015.

Berber, Eren. "Complications of Hypothyroidism." Endocrine Web. Accessed May 15, 2016. www.endocrineweb.com/ conditions/hypothyroidism/complications-hypothyroidism.

Childs, Westin. *Hashimoto's Diet Guide: How to Heal Your Thyroid and Boost Your Metabolism with the Thyroid Reset Diet.* Amazon Digital Services, 2015. Kindle edition.

"Eating with Hashimoto's Disease." The Science of Eating. Accessed May 15, 2016. http://thescienceofeating.com/food-combining-how-it-works/eating-with-hashimotos-disease.

Frazier, Karen. *The Hashimoto's Cookbook and Action Plan: 31 Days to Eliminate Toxins and Restore Thyroid Health through Diet.* Berkeley, CA: Rockridge Press, 2015.

"Hashimoto's Disease." National Institute of Diabetes and Digestive and Kidney Diseases. Accessed May 15, 2016. www .niddk.nih.gov/health-information/health-topics/endocrine/ hashimotos-disease/Pages/fact-sheet.aspx.

Hedberg, Nikolas, and Danielle Cook. *The Complete Thyroid Health and Diet Guide: Understanding and Managing Thyroid Disease.* Toronto, ON: Robert Rose, 2015.

Hedberg, Nikolas Robert. *The Thyroid Alternative*. Renew Your Health, 2011.

"How to Boost Your Immune System." Harvard Health Publications. Accessed May 15, 2016. www.health.harvard.edu/staying-healthy/how-to-boost-your-immune-system.

Milas, Kresimira. "Hashimoto's Thyroiditis Overview." Endocrine Web. Accessed May 15, 2016. www.endocrineweb.com/conditions/hashimotos-thyroiditis/hashimotos-thyroiditis-overview/.

Myers, Amy. *The Autoimmune Solution: Prevent and Reverse the Full Spectrum of Inflammatory Symptoms and Diseases*. New York: Harper Collins Publishers, 2015.

Pick, Marcelle. "Goitrogens and Thyroid Health—The Good News!" Women to Women. Accessed May 15, 2016. www.womentowomen.com/thyroid-health/goitrogens-and-thyroid-health-the-good-news.

Ryan, Marc. "Hashimoto's Is an Autoimmune Disease, So Why Is Everyone Ignoring the Autoimmune Part?" Hashimoto's Healing. Accessed May 15, 2016. www.hashimotoshealing.com/hashimotos-is-an-autoimmune-disease-so-why-is-everyone-ignoring-the-autoimmune-part.

"Thyroid Information." American Thyroid Association. Accessed May 15, 2016. www.thyroid.org/thyroid-information.

Zimmerman, Kim Ann. "Endocrine System: Facts, Functions and Diseases." LiveScience. Accessed March 11, 2016. www.livescience.com/26496-endocrine-system.html.

GENERAL INDEX

INDEX OF RECIPES

ABOUT THE AUTHOR

Kate Barrington graduated from Marietta College in 2009 with a Bachelor's Degree in English and a creative writing concentration. Since then she has obtained an ISSA Fitness Nutrition Coach certification and has built a business for herself as a freelance writer specializing in health and fitness niche topics. Kate uses her combined education and professional experience to craft original recipes for cookbooks and to create in-depth diet guides. She is also an animal lover and a regular contributor for several pet magazines and major pet websites.